# *Does My BUTT Look Big In This BEER?*
## *Nutritional Values of 2,000 Worldwide Beers*

## — Bob Skilnik —
### aka, The Low-Carb Bartender

Pick up a candy bar, a bag of potato chips, or even your kid's favorite sugar-coated breakfast cereals and you can refer to a Nutrition Facts label that gives you the kind of nutritional information that you, the consumer, deserves to know.

**But pick up a bottle or can of your favorite beer, and unless it's a low-calorie or low-carbohydrate brew with a federally-required Nutrition Facts label emblazoned on it, you have no idea what, if any, nutritional components are in a regular-brewed stout, porter, bock, wheat beer or even a simple American-style pilsner beer...**

...**Until NOW!** Whether you're counting calories, carbs or even Weight Watchers® Points®, here's a compilation of the nutritional information that you can't find anywhere else but in these following pages for **<u>over 2,000 worldwide beers.</u>**

## *Moderation, Not Deprivation!*

# Also by Bob Skilnik

*The Low-Carb Bartender:*
*Carb Counts For Beer, Wine, Mixed*
*Drinks And More*

*The Drink Beer, Get Thin Diet:*
*A Low-Carbohydrate Approach*

*101 Ways To Cut Fats And Carbs*

# Does My BUTT Look BIG In This BEER?

*Nutritional Values of
2,000 Worldwide Beers*

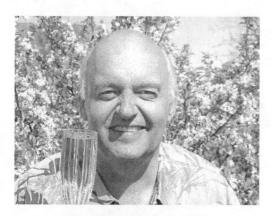

## Bob Skilnik

# Gambrinus Media
## Plainfield, IL

ISBN-10: 0-9822182-0-6

ISBN-13: 978-0-9822182-0-4

This book is printed on acid free paper.


Library of Congress Control Number: 2008911844

Library of Congress subject headings:

Health & Fitness: Diets – Better Health

Health & Fitness: Diets – Special Conditions

Health & Fitness: Nutrition

WEIGHT WATCHERS® and POINTS® are registered trademarks of Weight Watchers International, Inc. The number of POINTS® provided here was calculated based on published Weight Watchers International, Inc., information and does not imply sponsorship or endorsement of such number of POINTS® or products by Weight Watchers International, Inc.

Please note: The following information is provided as a general guide of various beers and their nutritional values. It is not a substitute for specific advice from your General Practitioner. The contents of this book are for informational and entertainments purposes only and are meant to be discussed with your physician or other qualified health care professional before being acted on. Never disregard any advice given to you by your doctor or other qualified health care professional. Always seek the advice of a physician or other licensed health care professional regarding any questions you have about your medical condition(s) and treatment(s). **This book is not a substitute for medical advice.**

## Acknowledgements

Information for the nutritional content of beers listed in the book was graciously provided by many worldwide breweries who understand that an informed customer is a repeat customer. As a fellow beer drinker, I ask that you please patronize them and enjoy their products as they helped make this book possible.

Last, but not least, a continuing thanks to my wife, Daria, who wants me to write *The Great American Novel*, make millions and retire to the south of France, but instead puts up with my incessant writing about all things beer, wine and booze related.

# All New In 2009
# From
# <u>Gambrinus Media</u>

## *The ALL NEW Drink Beer, Get Thin Diet*

### *&*

## *The Smart Drinkers Nutritional Guide for Beer, Wine and Booze:*

### *With 101 Healthy and Satisfying Recipes of Your Favorite Adult Drinks*

# Contents

# Serving Facts

| Serving Size | 12 fl oz (355 ml) |
| Servings Per Container | 1 |

| | Amount Per Serving |
| --- | --- |
| **Alcohol by volume** | 4% |
| fl oz of alcohol | 0.5 |
| **Calories** | 90 |
| **Carbohydrate** | 2g |
| **Fat** | 0g |
| **Protein** | 1g |

DEPARTMENT OF THE TREASURY

Alcohol and Tobacco Tax and Trade Bureau

**Federal Register** / Vol. 72, No. 146 / Tuesday, July 31, 2007 /
Proposed Rules

# Preface

Whether brewers, vintners or distillers like it or not, the Alcohol Tobacco Tax and Trade Bureau (TTB), responsible for labeling requirements of alcoholic beverages, is close to making it mandatory for alcoholic beverages to list their nutritional values. When the TTB finally arrives at some sort of standardized Nutrition Facts label that makes sense (it might take years), they have assured the drink industry that once they settle on an idea of what will be needed on the Nutrition Facts label, they will still give industry members an additional three years to redesign new labels and ease the cost of testing and relabeling by gradually implementing their compliance timeline.

One compelling reason why this will come to fruition is because of the hand of globalism in today's universal trade and commerce. As the Distilled Spirits Council of the United States notes in their most recent comment in TTB Notice No. 74, *"...this proposed rule change would bring TTB requirements into conformity with the provisions of the World Wine Trade Group (WWTG) Agreement on Wine Labelling. As stated by TTB, '[these] negotiations proceeded from the view that common labeling requirements would provide industry members with the opportunity to use the same label when shipping product to each of the WWTG member countries. With a global economy and with free travel among consumers, we support TTB's effort to harmonize its labeling regulations with international requirements. **TTB's proposal would have the beneficial effect of serving the interests of consumers, as well as <u>eliminating a potential barrier to trade between countries</u>.**'"*

Change is coming and it has the tailwinds of consumer support and NAFTA-inspired conformity behind it with a soon-to-be standardized world market of beer, wine and booze labels. Without acceptance by U.S. drink manufacturers, it's conceivable that the import/export markets of beers, wines and spirits would come to a halt; but be assured, that that will not happen.

So in reality, the global economy and the high costs of different drink labels for different world markets are probably more the driving forces behind the eventuality of nutritional labeling on beer, wine and booze than any concerns about the wants or needs of consumers. You know who will win this battle.

But why worry about any of this? In the following pages, you'll find nutritional information *now* that will help you to enjoy the moderate consumption of worldwide beer whether you're counting calories, carbohydrates or WEIGHT WATCHERS® POINTS®, perhaps even trying to pack on the pounds, or simply trying to maintain your current weight. You can even use the alcohol by volume (abv) information in this reference guide to settle bar bets; *What's the strongest beer? The weakest?*, for instance.

## TTB Measurement Tolerances

*"The Bureau [TTB] has determined that tolerance ranges are required with respect to labeled statements of caloric, carbohydrate, protein, and fat contents for malt beverages. The intent of these tolerances is to provide for normal production and analytical variables while continuing to ensure that the labeling is not misleading to the consumer.*

*Held, the statement of caloric content on labels for malt beverages will be considered acceptable as long as the caloric content, as determined by ATF [Alcohol Tobacco and Firearms Bureau] analysis, is within the tolerance +5 and -10 calories of the labeled caloric content. For example a label showing 96 calories will be acceptable if ATF analysis of the product shows a caloric content between 86 and 101 calories.*

*Held further, the statements of carbohydrate and fat contents on labels for malt beverages will be considered acceptable as long as the carbohydrate and fat contents, as determined by ATF analysis, are within a reasonable range below the labeled amount but, in no case, are more than 20% above the labeled amount. For example, a label showing 4.0 grams (within good manufacturing practice limitations) but not more than 4.8 grams.*

*Held further, the statement of protein content on labels for malt beverages will be considered acceptable as long as the protein content, as determined by ATF analysis, is within a reasonable range above the labeled amount but, in no case, is less than 80% of the labeled amount. For example, a label showing 1.0 gram protein will be acceptable if ATF analysis of the product shows a protein content which is more than 1.0 gram (within good manufacturing practice limitations) but no less than 0.8 gram."*

## Book Guidelines

You'll probably notice disparities between the nutritional information for the same brands of beer, but brewed in different countries. *Guinness* or *Beck's* comes to mind. Some worldwide breweries contract to have their beers brewed in satellite breweries, far from their home offices. The use of more easily available indigenous grains or accommodating known taste preferences of local beer drinkers can influence the use of different mixtures of grains in the mash, differently treated water sources, changing ratios of various types of hops in the kettle, and even yeast strains in the fermentor, which can account for variances in calories, carbohydrates and alcohol levels for the same brand of beers in different countries. *Guinness*, for instance, is extremely popular in Nigeria, yet the cost of shipping malted barley from Ireland would be prohibitive. As a result, indigenous grains such as sorghum and soybeans can also be added to the grain bill. As noted throughout the book, and reflective of different brewing practices in a host of countries, the nutritional values for *Guinness* will vary widely.

Serving size for beer is listed in the book as 12-ounces (with rare exceptions), even if the beer comes in 22-ounce "bombers" or half-liter bottles, as per the TTB and the United States Department of Agriculture (USDA) suggestions. That serving size (12-ounces) for beer will assuredly be solidified when the TTB makes its final decision on labeling requirements. I have no idea how the TTB will handle high-strength beers such as The Boston Beer Company's *Utopia* or *Millenium* brands, for instance. The brewery recommends a moderate 2-ounce serving size for these high-alcohol brews, but with a standardized beer serving being defined as 12-ounces, this is just one more problem that the TTB will have to deal with.

No sodium, fat, cholesterol or protein values are listed here. **There is NO fat nor cholesterol in beer** and trace amounts of sodium and protein values in your favorite brew. While TTB mandated alcoholic drink labels will almost assuredly display protein levels in grams and sodium levels in milligrams—all part of a labeling consistency for beer, wine, liquor and liqueurs—these numbers in beer are insignificant in my opinion, especially in light of the government recommendation of **no more than two 12-ounce servings of beer for men and one 12-ounce serving of suds for women per day**. For instance, the United States Department of Agriculture's *Recommended Dietary Allowance* (RDA) for sodium for a 25 old male is 1500 mg. Your average 12-ounce serving of *Budweiser* contains less than 10 mg of sodium. The average 12-ounce serving of *Budweiser* also contains 1.3 grams (gm) of protein while the RDA for protein for a male, 25 years and older, is 63 grams. (I used a 25-year old male for obvious reasons; they do enjoy their beers.) You could check out similar parameters for 25-year old women or different ages for men and women and you'd never find any beer, let alone a *Budweiser*, coming anywhere near RDA levels. You'd have to drink more than 150 bottles of *Budweiser* to hit the sodium RDA or chug down a little more than 49 bottles of the stuff to hit the protein RDA. Remember again; we're considering the fed's recommendation of no more than two 12-ounce servings of beer a day for men and one serving for women. The need to worry about sodium and protein in beer seems like a wasted exercise, so these nutritional values are ignored here.

One more caveat. Breweries are changing, and tweaking their recipes all the time, skewing their beers' nutritional values with any given batch. Also be aware that any measurement of the nutritional values of beer is based on an **average analysis**. No two batches of beer will ever be the same. That's why the TTB gives an expected range (+, -) for calorie, carbohydrate and protein analyses. Of the many breweries that contributed to this book, The Lion Brewery in Wilkes-Barre, Pennsylvania was the only brewery that sent me their beer nutritional information with *expected ranges*, not as definitive numbers. That's really how you have to look at the information in this book; numbers will fluctuate with each batch of beer. Keeping the nutritional data within an expected range and deriving an **average analysis** of product is what's given here.

**I welcome any documented corrections and additions to the material presented here and will post them on our website and will also include the newest numbers in future printings of this book.** There are more than 2,000 beers in this list, the majority of them with ALL their carbs, calories, and alcohol by volume percentages listed. You'll waste your time going through the various websites with nutritional values of beer. Using info direct from the breweries, I've often found that the website nutritional values are wrong; more often than not, very wrong!

This material, as presented, is copyrighted. Slight "ringers" with an insignificant difference of .01 g carbs or 1 calorie have been added to the list to track any attempts to duplicate this material.

We'll be online with ever-expanding information on beer, wine, and booze nutritional values and be presenting plenty of tips on how to enjoy all of them in a moderate, responsible and healthful manner.   http://MyBeerButt.com

On the website, you'll find:

- New and updated information  for the nutritional values for beer, wine and booze as more numbers come in
- Lower-calorie, lower-carbohydrate and lower-fat recipe versions of your favorite mixed-drinks
- Tasty recipes for making your own lower-calorie, lower-carbohydrate and lower-fat liquors, liqueurs and bar mixes
- Food recipes using beer, wine and booze as condiments, with an emphasis on flavorful and healthy dishes
- Video presentations of much of what's listed above
- A drink recipe exchange forum

|  | Oz | Carbs | Cal | Abv | Weight Watcher's POINTS® |
|---|---|---|---|---|---|
| **23rd Street** | | | | | |
| Bitter Professor | 12 | 19.00 | 182 | 05.50 | 4 |
| Chrimson Phog Irish Ale | 12 | 18.40 | 200 | 06.50 | 4 |
| Larryville Lyte | 12 | 14.60 | 158 | 05.25 | 3 |
| Little Dublin Dry Stout | 12 | 15.70 | 173 | 05.70 | 3 |
| Raspberry Wheat | 12 | 14.30 | 173 | 05.00 | 3 |
| Wave the Wheat | 12 | 14.30 | 153 | 05.00 | 3 |
| **Abita** | | | | | |
| Amber | 12 | 10.00 | 128 | 04.50 | 2 |
| Andygator | 12 | 19.00 | 235 | 07.75 | 5 |
| Bock | 12 | 16.00 | 187 | 06.50 | 4 |
| Christmas Ale (varies year to year) | 12 | 12.00 | | 05.00 | |
| Fall Fest | 12 | 15.00 | 167 | 05.40 | 3 |
| Golden | 12 | 10.00 | 125 | 04.20 | 2 |
| Jockamo IPA | 12 | 13.00 | 190 | 06.50 | 4 |
| Light | 12 | 08.00 | 118 | 04.00 | 2 |
| Pecan Harvest | 12 | 11.00 | 150 | 05.00 | 3 |
| Purple Haze | 12 | 11.00 | 128 | 04.20 | 2 |
| Red Ale | 12 | 11.00 | 151 | 05.20 | 3 |
| Restoration Ale | 12 | 15.00 | 167 | 04.90 | 3 |
| Strawberry | 12 | 11.00 | 128 | 04.20 | 2 |
| Turbo Dog | 12 | 16.00 | 168 | 05.60 | 3 |
| Stout | 12 | 19.75 | 167 | 04.50 | 3 |
| Wheat | 12 | 10.00 | 125 | 04.20 | 2 |

|  | Oz | Carbs | Cal | Abv | Weight Watcher's POINTS® |
|---|---|---|---|---|---|
| **Alaskan** | | | | | |
| Amber (Alt) | 12 | 18.20 | 184 | 05.30 | 4 |
| BW 2004 | 12 | 44.70 | 373 | 10.40 | 7 |
| ESB | 12 | 18.20 | 197 | 05.30 | 4 |
| IPA | 12 | 16.00 | 210 | 06.20 | 4 |
| Pale | 12 | 13.60 | 160 | 05.20 | 3 |
| Smoked Porter | 12 | 22.50 | 225 | 06.50 | 4 |
| Summer Ale | 12 | 13.40 | 184 | 05.30 | 4 |
| Oatmeal Stout | 12 | 24.10 | 225 | 05.70 | 4 |
| Winter Ale | 12 | 24.10 | 225 | 06.40 | 4 |
| **Alley Kat (Canada)** | | | | | |
| Amber | 12 | 16.00 | 159 | 05.00 | 3 |
| Aprikat | 12 | 12.10 | 120 | 04.10 | 2 |
| Full Moon | 12 | 14.75 | 156 | 05.00 | 3 |
| Scona Gold | 12 | 13.00 | 150 | 05.00 | 3 |
| **Allagash** | | | | | |
| 11th Anniversary | 12 | 28.70 | 293 | 09.20 | 6 |
| Black | 12 | 23.10 | 237 | 07.50 | 5 |
| Curieux | 12 | 15.90 | 257 | 10.00 | 5 |
| Dubbel | 12 | 18.50 | 209 | 07.00 | 4 |
| Fluxus | 12 | 16.20 | 233 | 08.70 | 5 |
| Fluxus '07 | 12 | 20.40 | 275 | 10.00 | 5 |
| Fluxus '08 | 12 | 16.20 | 233 | 08.70 | 5 |
| Four | 12 | 25.00 | 293 | 10.00 | 6 |
| Grand Cru | 12 | 20.10 | 220 | 07.20 | 4 |
| Hugh Malone | 12 | 24.30 | 262 | 08.50 | 5 |
| Interlude | 12 | 18.90 | 259 | 09.50 | 5 |
| Musette | 12 | 21.30 | 279 | 10.00 | 5 |

| | Oz | Carbs | Cal | Abv | Weight Watcher's POINTS® |
|---|---|---|---|---|---|
| Odyssey | 12 | 19.00 | 277 | 10.40 | 5 |
| Tripel | 12 | 19.80 | 253 | 09.00 | 5 |
| Victor Ale | 12 | 19.00 | 277 | 10.40 | 5 |
| Victoria Ale | 12 | 21.80 | 261 | 09.00 | 5 |
| White | 12 | 15.30 | 159 | 05.00 | 3 |

## Alpine

| | Oz | Carbs | Cal | Abv | Weight Watcher's POINTS® |
|---|---|---|---|---|---|
| Ale | 12 | 11.25 | 155 | 05.50 | 3 |
| Captain Stout | 12 | 17.00 | 177 | 05.60 | 3 |
| Duet | 12 | 20.50 | 213 | 06.75 | 4 |
| Mandarin Nectar | 12 | 09.25 | 166 | 06.50 | 3 |
| Mcllenney's Irish Red | 12 | 13.25 | 172 | 06.10 | 3 |
| Pure Hoppiness | 12 | 20.25 | 240 | 08.10 | 5 |
| Willy | 12 | 07.50 | 131 | 05.00 | 3 |
| Willy Vanilly | 12 | 07.50 | 131 | 05.00 | 3 |

## Alpirsbacher Klosterbrauerei (Germany)

| | Oz | Carbs | Cal | Abv | Weight Watcher's POINTS® |
|---|---|---|---|---|---|
| Spezial | 12 | 15.95 | 166 | 05.02 | 3 |
| Pils | 12 | 15.45 | 155 | 04.80 | 3 |
| Kloster Dunkel | 12 | 15.95 | 166 | 05.20 | 3 |
| Light | 12 | 09.60 | 094 | 02.09 | 2 |
| Kloster Weisse Dunkel | 12 | 13.20 | 154 | 05.20 | 3 |
| Kloster Wesse Hefetrub | 12 | 18.65 | 174 | 05.02 | 3 |
| Kloster Krystalklar | 12 | 13.20 | 154 | 05.20 | 3 |

## Amstel (Holland)

| | Oz | Carbs | Cal | Abv | Weight Watcher's POINTS® |
|---|---|---|---|---|---|
| Amstel | 12 | 10.65 | 142 | 05.00 | 3 |
| Bock | 12 | 17.75 | 213 | 07.00 | 4 |
| Gold | 12 | 14.20 | 213 | 07.00 | 4 |

| | Oz | Carbs | Cal | Abv | Weight Watcher's POINTS® |
|---|---|---|---|---|---|
| Lentebock | 12 | 17.74 | 213 | 07.00 | 4 |
| Light | 12 | 05.33 | 089 | 03.50 | 2 |
| Meibock | 12 | 17.75 | 213 | 07.00 | 4 |
| Malt | 12 | 21.30 | 089 | 00.10 | 2 |
| Oud Bruin | 12 | 19.52 | 124 | 02.50 | 2 |
| 1870 | 12 | 12.42 | 160 | 05.00 | 3 |

## Anchor

| | Oz | Carbs | Cal | Abv | Weight Watcher's POINTS® |
|---|---|---|---|---|---|
| Anchor Porter | 12 | 23.53 | 209 | 05.60 | 4 |
| Anchor Steam | 12 | 16.00 | 155 | 04.90 | 3 |
| Liberty Ale | 12 | | 188 | 06.00 | 4 |

## Andechs (Germany)

| | Oz | Carbs | Cal | Abv | Weight Watcher's POINTS® |
|---|---|---|---|---|---|
| Bergbock Hell | 12 | | 142 | 07.00 | 3 |
| Dopplebock Dunkel | 12 | | 156 | 07.00 | 3 |
| Dunkel | 12 | | 104 | 05.10 | 2 |
| Dunkles Weissbier | 12 | | 111 | 05.00 | 2 |
| Helles | 12 | | 106 | 04.80 | 2 |
| Spezial Helles | 12 | | 116 | 05.80 | 2 |
| Weissbier | 12 | | 106 | 05.00 | 2 |

## Anderson Valley

| | Oz | Carbs | Cal | Abv | Weight Watcher's POINTS® |
|---|---|---|---|---|---|
| Barney Flats Oatmeal Stout | 12 | 22.30 | 204 | 05.80 | 4 |
| Boont ESB | 12 | 16.30 | 182 | 05.90 | 4 |
| Brother David's Double | 12 | 21.70 | 255 | 08.70 | 5 |
| Brother David's Triple | 12 | 21.60 | 285 | 10.30 | 6 |
| Deependers Dark Porter | 12 | 15.30 | 170 | 05.50 | 3 |
| High Rollers Wheat | 12 | 13.40 | 157 | 05.30 | 3 |

| | Oz | Carbs | Cal | Abv | Weight Watcher's POINTS® |
|---|---|---|---|---|---|
| Hop Ottin' IPA | 12 | 17.80 | 211 | 07.20 | 4 |
| Poleeko Gold Pale | 12 | 14.00 | 163 | 05.50 | 3 |
| Summer Solstice | 12 | 16.40 | 174 | 05.60 | 3 |
| Winter Solstice Seasonal Ale | 12 | 17.60 | 205 | 06.90 | 4 |

## Andreas (Germany)

| | Oz | Carbs | Cal | Abv | Weight Watcher's POINTS® |
|---|---|---|---|---|---|
| Pils | 12 | | 138 | 04.90 | 3 |

## Anheuser-Busch

All A-B products have an average 9 mg of sodium per 12 oz. serving. This is considered "very low" in sodium content by the Food and Drug Administration (FDA) definition.

| | Oz | Carbs | Cal | Abv | Weight Watcher's POINTS® |
|---|---|---|---|---|---|
| 180 High Energy Drink | 8.2 | 33.00 | 120 | 00.00 | 2 |
| 180 Orange Energy Drink Sugar-Free | 8.2 | 01.00 | 005 | 00.00 | 0 |
| 180 – Blue Energy Drink | 8.2 | 31.00 | 120 | 00.00 | 2 |
| 180 – Blue Energy Drink Low-Calorie | 8.2 | 04.00 | 015 | 00.00 | 0 |
| 180 – Red Energy Drink | 8.2 | 32.00 | 130 | 00.00 | 3 |
| Anheuser World Lager | 12 | 14.50 | 165 | 05.00 | 3 |
| Bacardi Silver Big Apple | 12 | 36.30 | 240 | 05.00 | 5 |
| Bacardi Silver Mojito | 12 | 33.50 | 229 | 05.00 | 4 |
| Bacardi Silver Strawberry | 12 | 36.30 | 240 | 05.00 | 5 |
| Bacardi Silver Raz | 12 | 36.30 | 240 | 05.00 | 5 |
| Bacardi Silver O3 | 12 | 36.30 | 240 | 05.00 | 5 |
| Bacardi Silver Watermelon | 12 | 36.30 | 240 | 05.00 | 5 |

| | Oz | Carbs | Cal | Abv | Weight Watcher's POINTS® |
|---|---|---|---|---|---|
| Bacardi Silver Peach | 12 | 36.30 | 240 | 05.00 | 5 |
| Bare Knuckle Stout | 12 | 07.30 | 110 | 04.20 | 2 |
| Beach Bum Blonde Ale | 12 | 12.90 | 163 | 05.40 | 3 |
| Budweiser | 12 | 10.60 | 145 | 05.00 | 3 |
| Budweiser American Ale | 12 | 16.50 | 177 | 05.30 | 3 |
| Budweiser 3.2 | 12 | 08.70 | 116 | 04.00 | 2 |
| Budweiser Select | 12 | 03.10 | 099 | 04.30 | 2 |
| Bud Light | 12 | 06.60 | 110 | 04.20 | 2 |
| Bud Light 3.2 | 12 | 05.20 | 105 | 03.95 | 2 |
| Bud Light Lime | 12 | 08.00 | 116 | 03.10 | 2 |
| Bud Ice | 12 | 03.80 | 123 | 05.50 | 2 |
| Bud Ice Light | 12 | 06.50 | 110 | 04.00 | 2 |
| Bud Ice Light 3.2 | 12 | 03.60 | 109 | 04.04 | 2 |
| Bud Dry | 12 | 07.80 | 130 | 05.00 | 3 |
| Bud Dry 3.2 | 12 | 06.30 | 105 | 03.95 | 2 |
| Chelada Budweiser | 12 | 20.30 | 186 | 05.00 | 4 |
| Chelada Bud Light | 12 | 15.60 | 151 | 04.20 | 3 |
| Doc's Hard Lemon | 12 | 16.50 | | | |
| IntensiTea Peach | 12 | 27.40 | 217 | 05.50 | 4 |
| IntensiTea Lemon | 12 | 27.40 | 217 | 05.50 | 4 |
| IntensiTea Raspberry | 12 | 27.40 | 217 | 05.50 | 4 |
| Jack's Pumpkin Spice | 12 | 16.00 | 175 | 05.50 | 3 |
| Killarney's | 12 | 21.90 | 200 | 05.00 | 4 |
| Michelob | 12 | 15.00 | 164 | 05.00 | 3 |
| Michelob 3.2 | 12 | 12.20 | 124 | 03.95 | 2 |

| | Oz | Carbs | Cal | Abv | Weight Watcher's POINTS® |
|---|---|---|---|---|---|
| Michelob Light | 12 | 08.80 | 123 | 04.30 | 2 |
| Michelob Light 3.2 | 12 | 09.30 | 112 | 03.55 | 2 |
| Michelob Ultra | 12 | 02.60 | 095 | 04.20 | 2 |
| Michelob Ultra Amber | 12 | 03.70 | 114 | 05.00 | 2 |
| Michelob Ultra Lime Cactus | 12 | 06.00 | 107 | 04.20 | 2 |
| Michelob Ultra Pomegranate Raspberry | 12 | 06.00 | 107 | 04.20 | 2 |
| Michelob Ultra Tuscan Orange | 12 | 06.00 | 107 | 04.20 | 2 |
| Michelob Golden Draft | 12 | 14.10 | 152 | 04.70 | 3 |
| Michelob Golden Draft 3.2 | 12 | 10.50 | 129 | 04.00 | 2 |
| Michelob Golden Draft Light | 12 | 06.60 | 110 | 04.10 | 2 |
| Michelob Golden Draft Light 3.2 | 12 | 05.50 | 107 | 04.00 | 2 |
| Michelob Amber Bock | 12 | 12.10 | 155 | 05.20 | 3 |
| Michelob Amber Bock 3.2 | 12 | 11.90 | 128 | 03.95 | 2 |
| Michelob Bavarian Wheat | 12 | 12.80 | 160 | 05.20 | 3 |
| Michelob Hefeweizen | 12 | 13.20 | 154 | 04.80 | 3 |
| Michelob Hefeweizen 3.2 | 12 | 11.90 | 132 | 03.95 | 3 |
| Michelob Maerzen | 12 | 16.20 | 172 | 05.10 | 3 |
| Michelob Porter | 12 | 13.20 | 180 | 05.10 | 4 |
| Michelob Pale Ale | 12 | 18.40 | 187 | 05.20 | 4 |

|  | Oz | Carbs | Cal | Abv | Weight Watcher's POINTS® |
|---|---|---|---|---|---|
| Michelob Honey Lager | 12 | 19.20 | 178 | 04.90 | 3 |
| Michelob Honey Lager 3.2 | 12 | 14.90 | 143 | 03.95 | 3 |
| Michelob Black & Tan | 12 | 16.30 | 171 | 05.00 | 3 |
| Michelob Ultra | 12 | 02.60 | 095 | 04.20 | 2 |
| Red Wolf | 12 | 11.70 | 158 | 05.40 | 3 |
| Red Wolf 3.2 | 12 | 09.20 | 114 | 03.95 | 2 |
| O'Doul's | 12 | 13.30 | 065 | 00.40 | 1 |
| O'Doul's Amber | 12 | 18.00 | 090 | 00.40 | 2 |
| Busch | 12 | 10.20 | 133 | 04.60 | 3 |
| Busch 3.2 | 12 | 08.10 | 114 | 03.90 | 2 |
| Busch NA | 12 | 12.90 | 060 | 00.40 | 1 |
| Busch Light | 12 | 03.20 | 095 | 04.10 | 2 |
| Busch Light 3.2 | 12 | 05.20 | 102 | 03.90 | 2 |
| Busch Ice | 12 | 12.50 | 171 | 05.90 | 3 |
| Busch Ice 3.2 | 12 | 10.30 | 114 | 03.90 | 2 |
| Harbin Lager | 12 | 11.20 | 144 | 04.60 | 3 |
| Kirin Ichiban | 12 | 12.10 | 147 | 05.00 | 3 |
| Kirin Light | 12 | 07.80 | 095 | 03.20 | 2 |
| Natural Light | 12 | 03.20 | 095 | 04.02 | 2 |
| Natural Light 3.2 | 12 | 05.30 | 098 | 03.90 | 2 |
| Natural Ice | 12 | 08.90 | 157 | 05.90 | 3 |
| Natural Ice 3.2 | 12 | 07.60 | 105 | 03.95 | 2 |
| King Cobra | 12 | 14.50 | 133 | 06.00 | 3 |
| Hurricane | 12 | 09.90 | 158 | 05.80 | 3 |
| Hurricane High Gravity | 12 | 06.70 | 188 | 08.10 | 4 |

| | Oz | Carbs | Cal | Abv | Weight Watcher's POINTS® |
|---|---|---|---|---|---|
| Hurricane Ice | 12 | 05.70 | 175 | 07.50 | 3 |
| Ray Hill's American Pilsner | 12 | 15.50 | 162 | 04.90 | 3 |
| Red Bridge | 12 | 16.40 | 160 | 04.80 | 3 |
| Shock Top | 12 | 14.80 | 168 | 05.20 | 3 |
| Tilt Green | 12 | 47.70 | 346 | 08.00 | 7 |
| Tilt Green Orange 4.0% ABV | 12 | 50.50 | 307 | 04.00 | 6 |
| Tlt Green Orange 6.0% ABV | 12 | 42.00 | 283 | 06.00 | 6 |
| Tlt Green Orange 6.6% ABV | 12 | 45.60 | 310 | 06.60 | 6 |
| Tequiza | 12 | 09.00 | 127 | 04.50 | 3 |
| Tequiza 3.2 | 12 | 08.10 | 112 | 04.00 | 2 |
| Winter's Bourbon Cask Ale | 12 | 10.20 | 165 | 06.00 | 3 |
| Zeigen Bock | 12 | 14.40 | 154 | 05.00 | 3 |
| Zeigen Bock Amber | 12 | 11.80 | 150 | 04.90 | 3 |

## Appalachian

| | Oz | Carbs | Cal | Abv | Weight Watcher's POINTS® |
|---|---|---|---|---|---|
| Abbey Roade Belgian | 12 | 18.50 | 203 | 06.70 | 4 |
| ABC ESB | 12 | 17.10 | 165 | 05.00 | 3 |
| Anniversary Maibock | 12 | 26.00 | 251 | 07.60 | 5 |
| Celtic Knot Red | 12 | 18.10 | 170 | 05.10 | 3 |
| Water Gap Wheat | 12 | 14.00 | 148 | 04.70 | 3 |
| Grinnin' Grizzly | 12 | 17.80 | 187 | 05.90 | 4 |
| Hinterland Hefe | 12 | 17.70 | 175 | 05.40 | 3 |
| Hoppy Trails IPA | 12 | 15.50 | 171 | 05.90 | 3 |
| Kipona Fest | 12 | 18.80 | 182 | 05.30 | 4 |

|  | Oz | Carbs | Cal | Abv | Weight Watcher's POINTS® |
|---|---|---|---|---|---|
| Mountain Lager | 12 | 15.40 | 154 | 04.50 | 3 |
| Pennypacker Porter | 12 | 19.50 | 188 | 05.50 | 4 |
| Peregrine Pilsner | 12 | 15.50 | 160 | 04.90 | 3 |
| Purist Pale Ale | 12 | 16.70 | 170 | 04.80 | 3 |
| Rockville Rye | 12 | 17.10 | 174 | 05.40 | 3 |
| Jolly Scot Ale | 12 | 19.00 | 182 | 05.30 | 4 |
| Sophie's Sparkling | 12 | 12.90 | 147 | 04.60 | 3 |
| Susquehanna Stout | 12 | 21.90 | 180 | 04.80 | 4 |
| Volks Weizenbock | 12 | 25.20 | 250 | 07.50 | 5 |
| Zoigl Star | 12 | 17.00 | 187 | 06.00 | 4 |

## Arbor

|  | Oz | Carbs | Cal | Abv | Weight Watcher's POINTS® |
|---|---|---|---|---|---|
| Bavarian Bliss Hefeweizen | 12 | 16.40 | 159 | 04.80 | 3 |
| Big Ben House Mild | 12 | 14.80 | 127 | 03.50 | 2 |
| Faricy Fest Irish Stout | 12 | 17.00 | 171 | 05.30 | 3 |
| Huxell Best Bitter | 12 | 15.50 | 139 | 04.00 | 3 |
| Jackhammer Old Ale | 12 | 27.40 | 264 | 08.00 | 5 |
| Milestone Porter | 12 | 20.70 | 217 | 06.90 | 4 |
| Olde Number 22 German Alt | 12 | 17.00 | 171 | 05.30 | 3 |
| Red Snapper Special Bitter | 12 | 16.40 | 159 | 04.80 | 3 |
| Sacred Cow IPA | 12 | 18.20 | 197 | 06.40 | 4 |
| Terminator Dopplebock | 12 | 28.80 | 299 | 09.30 | 6 |

|  | Oz | Carbs | Cal | Abv | Weight Watcher's POINTS® |
|---|---|---|---|---|---|
| **Arco Bräu (Germany)** | | | | | |
| Pilsener | 12 | 14.60 | 151 | 04.80 | 3 |
| Coronator | 12 | 27.80 | 258 | 07.60 | 5 |
| Leicht | 12 | 11.30 | 099 | 02.80 | 2 |
| Dunkel Weisse | 12 | 15.50 | 155 | 04.80 | 3 |
| Schloss Dunkel | 12 | 19.20 | 171 | 04.90 | 3 |
| Urweisse | 12 | 16.20 | 169 | 05.40 | 3 |
| Leicht Weisse | 12 | 10.50 | 099 | 02.09 | 2 |
| Urfass | 12 | 14.70 | 154 | 04.90 | 3 |
| Schloss Hell | 12 | 19.20 | 170 | 04.80 | 2 |
| **Ashai (Japan)** | | | | | |
| Super Dry | 12 | 10.30 | 146 | 04.80 | 3 |
| **August Schell** | | | | | |
| Light | 12 | 04.10 | 104 | 04.00 | 2 |
| Zommerfest | 12 | 13.70 | 152 | 05.00 | 3 |
| **Avery** | | | | | |
| 14'er ESB | 12 | 15.30 | 158 | 05.00 | 3 |
| Collaboration not Litigation Ale | 12 | 22.60 | 258 | 08.70 | 5 |
| Ellie's Brown | 12 | 19.50 | 185 | 05.50 | 4 |
| Fifteen | 12 | 15.00 | 207 | 07.70 | 4 |
| Fourteen | 12 | 27.70 | 292 | 09.50 | 6 |
| Hog Heaven | 12 | 25.00 | 278 | 09.20 | 5 |
| IPA | 12 | 17.20 | 190 | 06.30 | 4 |
| Karma | 12 | 14.10 | 157 | 05.20 | 3 |
| Mephistophele's | 12 | 30.40 | 434 | 16.10 | 9 |
| New World Porter | 12 | 21.30 | 214 | 06.70 | 4 |
| Old Jubilation | 12 | 21.90 | 242 | 08.00 | 5 |

| | Oz | Carbs | Cal | Abv | Weight Watcher's POINTS® |
|---|---|---|---|---|---|
| Out of Bounds | 12 | 20.00 | 179 | 05.10 | 4 |
| Redpoint | 12 | 18.50 | 172 | 05.10 | 3 |
| Salvation | 12 | 21.60 | 261 | 09.00 | 5 |
| Samael's Ale | 12 | 44.30 | 458 | 14.50 | 9 |
| The Beast | 12 | 40.60 | 480 | 16.40 | 10 |
| The Czar | 12 | 24.10 | 323 | 11.70 | 6 |
| The Kaiser | 12 | 19.70 | 259 | 09.37 | 5 |
| The Maharaja | 12 | 21.90 | 291 | 10.50 | 6 |
| The Reverend | 12 | 27.70 | 304 | 10.00 | 6 |
| Thirteen | 12 | 27.90 | 292 | 09.30 | 6 |
| White Rascal | 12 | 13.70 | 163 | 05.60 | 3 |
| **Ayinger (Germany)** | | | | | |
| Altbäririsch Dunkel | 12 | 18.50 | 171 | 05.00 | 3 |
| Bräu-Hell | 12 | 15.20 | 156 | 04.90 | 3 |
| Bräu-Weisse | 12 | 13.60 | 117 | 03.20 | 2 |
| Celebrator | 12 | 31.40 | 256 | 06.70 | 5 |
| Frühlingsbier | 12 | 15.80 | 170 | 05.80 | 3 |
| Jahrhundert Bier | 12 | 15.80 | 170 | 05.50 | 3 |
| Kellerbier | 12 | 15.20 | 156 | 04.90 | 3 |
| Kirta-Halbe | 12 | 18.00 | 184 | 05.80 | 4 |
| Premium Pils | 12 | 14.80 | 156 | 05.00 | 3 |
| Ur-Weisse | 12 | 16.70 | 180 | 05.80 | 4 |
| Winter-Bock | 12 | 31.40 | 256 | 06.70 | 5 |
| **Baltika (Russia)** | | | | | |
| Baltika Cooler | 12 | 12.00 | 150 | 04.70 | 3 |
| Baltika Dark Lager | 12 | 17.00 | 192 | 05.60 | 4 |
| Baltika N1 Light | 12 | 17.04 | 138 | 04.40 | 3 |

| | Oz | Carbs | Cal | Abv | Weight Watcher's POINTS® |
|---|---|---|---|---|---|
| Baltika N0 Non-alcoholic | 12 | 21.67 | 117 | <0.50 | 0 |
| Balitka N2 Pale | 12 | 12.07 | 146 | 04.70 | 3 |
| Baltika N3 Classic | 12 | 17.04 | 149 | 04.80 | 3 |
| Baltika N4 Original | 12 | 17.04 | 192 | 05.60 | 4 |
| Baltika N5 Gold | 12 | 10.65 | 158 | 05.30 | 3 |
| Baltika N6 Porter | 12 | 21.30 | 213 | 07.00 | 4 |
| Baltika N7 Export | 12 | 15.97 | 156 | 05.40 | 3 |
| Baltika N8 Wheat | 12 | 12.07 | 160 | 05.00 | 3 |
| Baltika N9 Extra | 12 | 13.14 | 220 | 08.00 | 4 |
| Baltika LITE | 12 | 12.43 | 131 | 04.00 | 3 |
| Don Zhivoye | 12 | 15.27 | 138 | 04.00 | 3 |
| DV Zhivoye | 12 | 16.69 | 153 | 04.40 | 3 |
| Leningradskoe Extra | 12 | 20.59 | 245 | 07.50 | 5 |
| Leningradskoe Lager | 12 | 15.62 | 153 | 04.00 | 3 |
| Medovoye (Honey) Light | 12 | 16.33 | 149 | 04.10 | 3 |
| Medovoye (Honey) Extra | 12 | 23.43 | 220 | 07.60 | 4 |
| Nevskoe ICE | 12 | 16.33 | 149 | 04.70 | 3 |
| Samara Classic | 12 | 13.49 | 165 | 05.00 | 3 |
| Samara Extra | 12 | 16.33 | 202 | 06.50 | 4 |
| Samara Zhivoye | 12 | 15.27 | 138 | 04.00 | 3 |
| Sibirskiy Bochonok Classic | 12 | 10.65 | 146 | 05.10 | 3 |
| Sibirskiy Bochonok Extra | 12 | 09.94 | 199 | 08.00 | 4 |
| Volga Yantarnoye Special | 12 | 16.69 | 163 | 05.00 | 3 |
| Yarpivo Extra | 12 | 20.59 | 192 | 07.20 | 4 |

|  | Oz | Carbs | Cal | Abv | Weight Watcher's POINTS® |
|---|---|---|---|---|---|
| Yarpivo Lager | 12 | 14.91 | 135 | 04.20 | 3 |
| Yarpivo Ledyanoe | 12 | 16.33 | 149 | 04.90 | 3 |
| Yarpivo Original | 12 | 16.33 | 149 | 04.70 | 3 |
| Yarpivo Yantarnoye | 12 | 16.69 | 163 | 05.30 | 3 |
| Zhigulevskoye | 12 | 16.33 | 149 | 04.00 | 3 |

## Baron

|  | Oz | Carbs | Cal | Abv | |
|---|---|---|---|---|---|
| Berliner-Weisse | 12 | 16.30 | 149 | 04.30 | 3 |
| Dampfbier | 12 | 17.60 | 172 | 05.20 | 3 |
| Doppelbock | 12 | 24.30 | 262 | 08.50 | 5 |
| Dunkel-Weisse | 12 | 17.10 | 165 | 05.00 | 3 |
| Hefe-Weisse | 12 | 17.10 | 165 | 05.00 | 3 |
| Helles Bock | 12 | 19.80 | 204 | 06.40 | 4 |
| Kristall-Weisse | 12 | 17.10 | 165 | 05.00 | 3 |
| Pilsner | 12 | 16.80 | 159 | 04.70 | 3 |
| Rauchbier | 12 | 15.30 | 158 | 05.00 | 3 |
| Roggen | 12 | 17.10 | 165 | 05.00 | 3 |
| Schwazbier | 12 | 16.60 | 162 | 04.90 | 3 |
| Über-Weisse | 12 | 23.50 | 253 | 08.20 | 5 |

## Bass (UK)

|  | Oz | Carbs | Cal | Abv | |
|---|---|---|---|---|---|
| Pale Ale | 12 | 13.20 | 132 | 05.00 | 3 |

## Bear Republic

|  | Oz | Carbs | Cal | Abv | |
|---|---|---|---|---|---|
| Big Bear Stout | 12 | 22.90 | 249 | 08.10 | 5 |
| English ESB | 12 | 21.90 | 181 | 04.80 | 4 |
| Heritage Ale | 12 | 26.90 | 255 | 07.60 | 5 |
| Hop Rod Rye | 12 | 24.90 | 244 | 07.50 | 5 |
| Late Harvest Fest Lager | 12 | 22.10 | 209 | 06.20 | 4 |
| Racer 5 | 12 | 24.00 | 231 | 07.00 | 5 |

|  | Oz | Carbs | Cal | Abv | Weight Watcher's POINTS® |
|---|---|---|---|---|---|
| Red Rocket | 12 | 22.40 | 221 | 06.80 | 4 |
| Special XP | 12 | 16.60 | 171 | 05.40 | 3 |
| Wine Country Wheat | 12 | 18.80 | 163 | 04.50 | 3 |

### Beck's (Germany)

|  | Oz | Carbs | Cal | Abv | Weight Watcher's POINTS® |
|---|---|---|---|---|---|
| Beck's | 12 | 10.00 | 138 | 05.00 | 3 |
| Beck's Dark | 12 | 11.00 | 146 | 04.80 | 3 |
| Beck's Light | 12 | 03.90 | 064 | 02.30 | 1 |
| Beck's Oktoberfest | 12 | 11.00 | 146 | 05.20 | 3 |
| Clausthaler Golden | 12 | 15.98 | 096 | 00.40 | 2 |
| Clausthaler Premium | 12 | 19.32 | 046 | 00.48 | 1 |
| Dribeck | 12 | 07.00 | 098 | 03.39 | 2 |
| Hacke Beck NA | 12 | 20.00 | 093 | 00.30 | 2 |
| St. Pauli Girl | 12 | 08.70 | 137 | 05.00 | 3 |
| St. Pauli Girl Dark | 12 | 08.70 | 150 | 04.80 | 3 |
| St. Pauli Girl NA | 12 | 23.00 | 096 | <0.50 | 2 |

### Bell's (See Kalamazoo)

### Big Sky

|  | Oz | Carbs | Cal | Abv | Weight Watcher's POINTS® |
|---|---|---|---|---|---|
| Moose Drool | 12 | 17.60 | 174 | 05.30 | 3 |

### Binding (Germany)

|  | Oz | Carbs | Cal | Abv | Weight Watcher's POINTS® |
|---|---|---|---|---|---|
| Doppelbock | 12 | 26.70 | 225 | 07.50 | 4 |
| Export | 12 | 15.10 | 160 | 05.30 | 3 |
| Guarana Verde | 12 | 30.90 | 195 | 04.00 | 4 |
| Kraft Malz | 12 | 39.70 | 165 | 00.30 | 3 |
| Lager | 12 | 11.90 | 135 | 04.50 | 3 |
| Römer Pils | 12 | 13.30 | 145 | 04.90 | 3 |
| Römer Pils Spezial | 12 | 13.00 | 145 | 05.00 | 3 |

| | Oz | Carbs | Cal | Abv | Weight Watcher's POINTS® |
|---|---|---|---|---|---|
| **Bitburger (Germany)** | | | | | |
| Bosman | 12 | | 160 | 06.20 | 3 |
| Drive NA | 12 | 20.59 | 103 | <0.50 | 2 |
| Kandi | 12 | 35.50 | 153 | 00.15 | 3 |
| Koestritzer | 12 | 09.94 | 146 | 04.80 | 3 |
| Light | 12 | 07.10 | 096 | 02.80 | 2 |
| Pils | 12 | 09.05 | 146 | 04.80 | 3 |
| Premium | 12 | 14.10 | 149 | 04.80 | 3 |
| **BJ's Restaurants** | | | | | |
| Brewhouse Blonde | 12 | 13.60 | 145 | 04.70 | 3 |
| Harvest Hefeweizen | 12 | 14.90 | 158 | 05.00 | 3 |
| Jeremiah Red Ale | 12 | 24.60 | 237 | 07.20 | 5 |
| Nutty Brewnette | 12 | 22.20 | 218 | 06.70 | 4 |
| Piranha Pale Ale | 12 | 17.00 | 187 | 06.00 | 4 |
| PM Porter | 12 | 21.90 | 216 | 06.60 | 4 |
| Tatonka Stout | 12 | 26.30 | 274 | 08.70 | 5 |
| **Blitz-Weinhard** | | | | | |
| Blue Boar | 12 | 12.40 | 144 | 04.60 | 3 |
| Classic Dark | 12 | | 169 | 04.81 | 3 |
| Hefeweizen | 12 | 12.90 | 151 | 04.86 | 3 |
| Northwest Trail | 12 | 14.10 | 161 | 05.12 | 3 |
| Summer Wheat | 12 | 13.30 | 153 | 04.90 | 3 |
| Private Reserve | 12 | 13.00 | 150 | 04.80 | 3 |
| **Blue Cat** | | | | | |
| Arkham Stout | 12 | 25.00 | 213 | 05.90 | 4 |
| Big Bad Dog Old Old English Ale | 12 | 25.60 | 226 | 06.40 | 4 |
| Blue Cat Porter | 12 | 19.90 | 170 | 04.70 | 3 |

| | Oz | Carbs | Cal | Abv | Weight Watcher's POINTS® |
|---|---|---|---|---|---|
| Count Magnus Dark Belgium Strong | 12 | 25.60 | 226 | 06.40 | 4 |
| Off the Rail Pale Ale | 12 | 16.70 | 165 | 05.10 | 3 |
| Wigged Pig Wheat | 12 | 13.40 | 158 | 05.30 | 3 |
| **Blue Mountain** | | | | | |
| BM Lager | 12 | 17.90 | 174 | 05.30 | 3 |
| Dubbel Ale | 12 | 28.90 | 265 | 07.70 | 5 |
| Pale Ale | 12 | 22.20 | 203 | 05.90 | 4 |
| Rockfish Wheat | 12 | 17.10 | 173 | 05.40 | 3 |
| **Boddington (UK)** | | | | | |
| Boddington | 12 | 12.78 | 197 | 04.80 | 4 |
| **Boston Beer Company** | | | | | |
| Black Lager | 12 | 23.90 | 191 | 04.90 | 4 |
| Brown Ale | 12 | 13.80 | 160 | 05.35 | 3 |
| Boston Ale | 12 | 19.90 | 180 | 05.10 | 4 |
| Boston Lager | 12 | 18.00 | 170 | 04.90 | 3 |
| Cherry Wheat | 12 | 16.86 | 180 | 05.40 | 4 |
| Chocolate Bock | 12 | 36.00 | 230 | 05.50 | 5 |
| Cranberry Lambic | 12 | 20.91 | 200 | 05.90 | 4 |
| Cream Stout | 12 | 23.94 | 190 | 04.90 | 4 |
| Double Bock | 12 | 32.40 | 310 | 08.80 | 6 |
| Golden Pilsner | 12 | 15.75 | 145 | 04.60 | 3 |
| Hallertau 24 | 12 | 18.50 | 169 | 05.10 | 3 |
| Hallertau Imperial Pilsner | 12 | 29.50 | 300 | 08.80 | 6 |
| Hefeweizen | 12 | 17.00 | 182 | 05.40 | 4 |
| Holiday Porter | 12 | 26.50 | 211 | 05.80 | 4 |
| Honey Porter | 12 | 20.57 | 192 | 05.45 | 4 |
| Irish Red | 12 | 20.00 | 180 | 05.50 | 4 |

|  | Oz | Carbs | Cal | Abv | Weight Watcher's POINTS® |
|---|---|---|---|---|---|
| Light | 12 | 09.70 | 119 | 04.05 | 2 |
| Millenium | 12 |  | 288 | 20.00 | 6 |
| Octoberfest | 12 | 18.72 | 180 | 05.40 | 3 |
| Old Fezziwig | 12 | 25.50 | 210 | 05.90 | 4 |
| Pale Ale | 12 | 13.40 | 160 | 05.40 | 3 |
| Scotch Ale | 12 | 24.96 | 200 | 05.40 | 4 |
| Summer Ale | 12 | 15.85 | 160 | 05.30 | 3 |
| Triple Bock | 12 |  | 636 | 18.00 | 12 |
| Utopia | 12 | 44.00 | 732 | 27.00 | 13+ |
| Winter Lager | 12 | 21.25 | 200 | 06.90 | 4 |

## Boulder Beer

|  | Oz | Carbs | Cal | Abv | Weight Watcher's POINTS® |
|---|---|---|---|---|---|
| Buffalo Gold | 12 | 18.70 | 167 | 04.95 | 3 |
| Pass Time | 12 | 19.00 | 173 | 05.00 | 3 |
| Planet Porter | 12 | 21.70 | 193 | 05.50 | 4 |
| Singletrack | 12 | 20.00 | 177 | 05.00 | 3 |
| Sundance | 12 | 18.70 | 168 | 04.85 | 3 |

## Boulevard

|  | Oz | Carbs | Cal | Abv | Weight Watcher's POINTS® |
|---|---|---|---|---|---|
| Bob's 47 | 12 | 18.50 | 185 | 05.50 | 4 |
| Bully Porter | 12 | 19.40 | 194 | 05.40 | 4 |
| Dry Stout | 12 | 14.70 | 149 | 04.90 | 3 |
| Irish Ale | 12 | 19.80 | 182 | 05.30 | 4 |
| Lunar | 12 | 18.80 | 157 | 04.50 | 3 |
| Nutcracker | 12 | 25.30 | 224 | 06.10 | 4 |
| Pale Ale | 12 | 15.80 | 163 | 05.10 | 3 |
| Unfiltered Wheat | 12 | 15.20 | 155 | 04.50 | 3 |
| Zōn | 12 | 14.10 | 153 | 04.40 | 3 |

|  | Oz | Carbs | Cal | Abv | Weight Watcher's POINTS® |
|---|---|---|---|---|---|
| **Bozeman** | | | | | |
| Hefe Weizen | 12 | 18.70 | 191 | 06.00 | 4 |
| Porter | 12 | 18.80 | 185 | 05.75 | 4 |
| Select | 12 | 16.30 | 171 | 05.50 | 3 |
| **Brahma (Brazil)** | | | | | |
| Chopp | 12 | | 152 | 05.00 | 3 |
| Chopp Claro | 12 | | 152 | 05.00 | 3 |
| Bock | 12 | | 185 | 05.90 | 4 |
| Escuro | 12 | | 183 | 06.00 | 4 |
| Extra | 12 | | 166 | 05.50 | 3 |
| Liber (NA) | 12 | | 088 | 00.00 | 2 |
| Light | 12 | | 094 | 03.10 | 2 |
| Malzbier | 12 | | 197 | 03.70 | 4 |
| **Brand (Holland)** | | | | | |
| Dubbelbock | 12 | 17.75 | 249 | 07.50 | 5 |
| Imperator | 12 | 14.20 | 213 | 06.50 | 4 |
| Meibock | 12 | 14.20 | 213 | 06.50 | 4 |
| Oud Bruin | 12 | 07.10 | 107 | 03.50 | 2 |
| Pilsner | 12 | 10.65 | 160 | 05.00 | 3 |
| Sylvester | 12 | 17.75 | 249 | 07.50 | 5 |
| UP | 12 | 12.43 | 160 | 05.50 | 3 |
| **BridgePort** | | | | | |
| Beertown Brown | 12 | 18.30 | 174 | 05.20 | 3 |
| Black Strap Stout | 12 | 25.60 | 218 | 06.00 | 4 |
| Blue Heron | 12 | 19.30 | 172 | 04.90 | 3 |
| Ebenezer | 12 | 23.30 | 217 | 06.40 | 4 |
| ESB | 12 | 20.20 | 199 | 06.10 | 4 |
| Haymaker | 12 | 17.00 | 171 | 05.30 | 3 |

| | Oz | Carbs | Cal | Abv | Weight Watcher's POINTS® |
|---|---|---|---|---|---|
| IPA | 12 | 18.60 | 181 | 05.50 | 4 |
| Old Knucklehead | 12 | 26.80 | 284 | 09.10 | 6 |
| Porter | 12 | 22.50 | 240 | 07.80 | 5 |
| Ropewalk | 12 | 17.40 | 179 | 05.60 | 3 |

### Bristol

| | Oz | Carbs | Cal | Abv | Weight Watcher's POINTS® |
|---|---|---|---|---|---|
| Beehive Honey Wheat | 12 | 16.20 | 155 | 04.60 | 3 |
| Laughing Lab Scottish Ale | 12 | 20.50 | 183 | 05.00 | 4 |
| Mass Transit Ale | 12 | 18.20 | 169 | 04.80 | 3 |
| Old No. 23 Barley Wine | 12 | 31.60 | 336 | 10.60 | 7 |
| Red Rocket Pale Ale | 12 | 15.75 | 159 | 05.10 | 3 |

### Brooklyn Brewery

| | Oz | Carbs | Cal | Abv | Weight Watcher's POINTS® |
|---|---|---|---|---|---|
| Brown Ale | 12 | 26.30 | 211 | 05.60 | 4 |
| East IPA | 12 | 21.30 | 181 | 06.80 | 4 |
| Lager | 12 | 28.40 | 170 | 05.20 | 3 |
| Pennant Pale | 12 | 23.90 | 191 | 05.00 | 4 |
| Weisse | 12 | 19.50 | 176 | 05.10 | 3 |

### Budejojovický Budvar (Czech)

| | Oz | Carbs | Cal | Abv | Weight Watcher's POINTS® |
|---|---|---|---|---|---|
| Premium Dark Lager | 12 | 15.85 | 153 | 04.70 | 3 |
| Premium Lager | 12 | 11.36 | 142 | 04.50 | 3 |

### Burleigh (Australia)

| | Oz | Carbs | Cal | Abv | Weight Watcher's POINTS® |
|---|---|---|---|---|---|
| Bighead | 12 | 00.00 | 088 | 04.20 | 2 |

### Butte Creek (Organic)

| | Oz | Carbs | Cal | Abv | Weight Watcher's POINTS® |
|---|---|---|---|---|---|
| IPA | 12 | 23.25 | 209 | 06.20 | 4 |
| Pale Ale | 12 | 19.50 | 166 | 05.10 | 3 |
| Pilsner | 12 | 15.50 | 154 | 04.40 | 3 |
| Porter | 12 | 22.50 | 184 | 05.50 | 4 |

|  | Oz | Carbs | Cal | Abv | Weight Watcher's POINTS® |
|---|---|---|---|---|---|

## Cambridge

|  | Oz | Carbs | Cal | Abv | Weight Watcher's POINTS® |
|---|---|---|---|---|---|
| Arquebus | 12 | 28.60 | 323 | 10.75 | 6 |
| Blackout Stout | 12 | 17.00 | 140 | 03.80 | 3 |
| Cambridge Amber | 12 | 16.40 | 159 | 04.80 | 3 |
| Charles River Porter | 12 | 19.80 | 198 | 06.10 | 4 |
| Great Pumpkin Ale | 12 | 15.80 | 146 | 04.20 | 3 |
| Gruit | 12 | 14.60 | 182 | 06.00 | 4 |
| Half-Wit | 12 | 13.50 | 144 | 04.70 | 3 |
| Hefe-Weizen | 12 | 13.70 | 163 | 05.50 | 3 |
| Heather Ale | 12 | 14.90 | 158 | 05.00 | 3 |
| Imperial Stout | 12 | 28.10 | 314 | 10.40 | 6 |
| Regatta Golden | 12 | 14.00 | 138 | 04.30 | 3 |
| Tall Tale Pale Ale | 12 | 18.70 | 191 | 06.00 | 4 |

## Captain Morgan (Malt-Based)

|  | Oz | Carbs | Cal | Abv | Weight Watcher's POINTS® |
|---|---|---|---|---|---|
| Parrot Bay Matava Blue | 12 | 37.30 | 241 | 05.00 | 5 |
| Parrot Bay Mojito | 12 | 37.60 | 234 | 05.00 | 5 |
| Parrot Bay Pineapple Coloada | 12 | 39.40 | 248 | 05.00 | 5 |
| Parrot Bay Sunset Surf | 12 | 39.80 | 248 | 05.00 | 5 |
| Parrot Bay Wave Runner | 12 | 39.40 | 248 | 05.00 | 5 |

## Carolina Beer & Beverage Company

|  | Oz | Carbs | Cal | Abv | Weight Watcher's POINTS® |
|---|---|---|---|---|---|
| Almond Stout | 12 |  | 200 | 06.00 | 4 |
| American Wheat | 12 |  | 155 | 05.30 | 3 |
| Blonde | 12 |  | 138 | 05.00 | 3 |
| Brown Ale | 12 |  | 170 | 05.70 | 3 |
| Endo IPA | 12 |  | 185 | 05.90 | 4 |

|  | Oz | Carbs | Cal | Abv | Weight Watcher's POINTS® |
|---|---|---|---|---|---|
| Frostbite | 12 |  | 250 | 09.00 | 5 |
| IPA | 12 |  | 170 | 05.90 | 3 |
| Irish Style Red | 12 |  | 150 | 04.50 | 3 |
| Lighthouse | 12 | 03.00 | 081 | 04.00 | 2 |
| Low Country Ale | 12 |  | 150 | 05.00 | 3 |
| Low Down Brown | 12 |  | 170 | 05.25 | 3 |
| Pumpkin Ale | 12 |  | 185 | 06.00 | 4 |
| Scottish Ale | 12 |  | 280 | 08.50 | 6 |
| Strawberry Ale | 12 |  | 135 | 04.75 | 3 |

### Carlsberg (Denmark)

|  | Oz | Carbs | Cal | Abv | Weight Watcher's POINTS® |
|---|---|---|---|---|---|
| Edge | 12 | 15.27 | 149 | 04.60 | 3 |
| Elephant Beer | 12 | 15.62 | 202 | 07.20 | 4 |
| Export | 12 | 09.94 | 149 | 05.00 | 3 |
| Lager | 12 | 07.10 | 114 | 03.80 | 2 |
| Light | 12 | 07.81 | 110 | 04.50 | 2 |
| Low-Alcohol | 12 | 10.65 | 057 | <0.50 | 1 |
| Mid-Strength | 12 | 11.36 | 107 | 02.60 | 2 |
| Special Brew | 12 | 18.82 | 249 | 09.00 | 5 |

### Cascade Lakes

|  | Oz | Carbs | Cal | Abv | Weight Watcher's POINTS® |
|---|---|---|---|---|---|
| 20" Brown | 12 | 17.90 | 175 | 05.30 | 3 |
| Blonde Bombshell | 12 | 12.10 | 131 | 04.00 | 3 |
| Bock | 12 | 22.10 | 224 | 07.00 | 4 |
| Imperial IPA | 12 | 26.40 | 276 | 08.80 | 5 |
| IPA | 12 | 19.80 | 198 | 06.10 | 4 |
| Kölsch | 12 | 14.80 | 148 | 04.60 | 3 |
| MacDougal's Amber | 12 | 17.30 | 178 | 05.50 | 3 |
| Monkey Face Porter | 12 | 18.50 | 172 | 05.00 | 3 |
| Pilsner | 12 | 15.20 | 148 | 04.50 | 3 |

| | Oz | Carbs | Cal | Abv | Weight Watcher's POINTS® |
|---|---|---|---|---|---|
| Pine Marten Pale Ale | 12 | 16.70 | 165 | 05.10 | 3 |
| Rooster Tail Ale | 12 | 15.15 | 164 | 05.30 | 3 |
| Santa's Little Helper | 12 | 21.90 | 212 | 06.40 | 4 |
| Weiss | 12 | 15.15 | 164 | 05.10 | 3 |

## Celis

| | Oz | Carbs | Cal | Abv | Weight Watcher's POINTS® |
|---|---|---|---|---|---|
| Grand Cru | 12 | 16.00 | 245 | 09.20 | 5 |

## Ceres (Denmark)

| | Oz | Carbs | Cal | Abv | Weight Watcher's POINTS® |
|---|---|---|---|---|---|
| Royal X-Mas Brew | 12 | 14.60 | 167 | 05.60 | 4 |

## Chimay (Belgium)

| | Oz | Carbs | Cal | Abv | Weight Watcher's POINTS® |
|---|---|---|---|---|---|
| White Triple | 12 | | 190 | 08.00 | 4 |

## Christian Moerlein

| | Oz | Carbs | Cal | Abv | Weight Watcher's POINTS® |
|---|---|---|---|---|---|
| Barbarossa | 12 | 23.50 | 191 | 05.00 | 4 |
| Emancipator | 12 | 25.80 | 239 | 07.00 | 5 |
| Golden Helles | 12 | 18.70 | 175 | 05.20 | 3 |
| OTR Ale | 12 | 26.90 | 224 | 06.00 | 4 |

## City Brewery

| | Oz | Carbs | Cal | Abv | Weight Watcher's POINTS® |
|---|---|---|---|---|---|
| City Lager | 12 | | 150 | 04.00 | 3 |
| City Light | 12 | | 115 | 03.40 | 2 |
| City Malt Liquor | 12 | | 156 | 04.60 | 3 |
| KUL | 12 | | 135 | 03.80 | 3 |
| KUL Lite | 12 | | 110 | 03.30 | 2 |
| La Crosse Lager | 12 | | 147 | 03.80 | 3 |
| La Crosse Light | 12 | | 112 | 03.30 | 2 |
| La Crosse NA | 12 | 12.00 | 060 | <0.50 | 1 |

## Cisco

| | Oz | Carbs | Cal | Abv | Weight Watcher's POINTS® |
|---|---|---|---|---|---|
| Sankaty Light | 12 | | 128 | 03.80 | 2 |

|  | Oz | Carbs | Cal | Abv | Weight Watcher's POINTS® |
|---|---|---|---|---|---|
| **Coast Range** | | | | | |
| California Blonde | 12 | 16.25 | 168 | 05.00 | 3 |
| Maduro Porter | 12 | 16.10 | 167 | 05.00 | 3 |
| Pale Ale | 12 | 20.00 | 183 | 05.20 | 4 |
| Scotch Ale | 12 | 31.00 | 267 | 06.90 | 5 |
| **Coastal Extreme** | | | | | |
| Alyssa | 12 | 19.00 | 228 | 07.90 | 4 |
| Brent | 12 | 18.00 | 240 | 08.40 | 5 |
| Chloe | 12 | 17.00 | 248 | 08.50 | 5 |
| Maelstrom IPA | 12 | 16.40 | 190 | 06.20 | 4 |
| Hurricane Amber | 12 | 12.30 | 150 | 05.20 | 3 |
| Irish Red | 12 | 13.10 | 150 | 05.10 | 3 |
| Oktoberfest | 12 | 20.20 | 192 | 05.30 | 4 |
| Porter | 12 | 20.20 | 192 | 05.50 | 4 |
| Spring Ale | 12 | 13.10 | 150 | 05.00 | 3 |
| Summer Ale | 12 | 16.40 | 190 | 06.20 | 4 |
| Winter Ale | 12 | 16.60 | 177 | 05.60 | 3 |
| **Cooper's (Australia)** | | | | | |
| Best Extra Stout | 12 | 10.65 | 181 | 06.30 | 4 |
| Birell | 12 | 14.73 | 075 | 00.50 | 1 |
| Dark Ale | 12 | 05.86 | 121 | 04.50 | 2 |
| Lager | 12 | 06.39 | 149 | 05.00 | 3 |
| Mild Ale | 12 | 05.33 | 142 | 03.50 | 3 |
| Original Pale Ale | 12 | 05.86 | 124 | 04.50 | 2 |
| Premium Lite | 12 | 04.44 | 092 | 02.90 | 2 |
| Sparkling Ale | 12 | 07.46 | 156 | 05.80 | 3 |
| Stout | 12 | 10.80 | 210 | 06.30 | 4 |

|  | Oz | Carbs | Cal | Abv | Weight Watcher's POINTS® |
|---|---|---|---|---|---|
| **Cooperstown** | | | | | |
| Old Slugger | 12 | 17.30 | 178 | 05.50 | 3 |
| Back Yard | 12 | 19.00 | 197 | 06.30 | 4 |
| Benchwarmer | 12 | 20.10 | 204 | 06.40 | 4 |
| Nine Man Ale | 12 | 15.90 | 149 | 04.30 | 3 |
| Pride of Milford | 12 | 19.70 | 227 | 07.70 | 4 |
| Strike Out Stout | 12 | 16.40 | 159 | 04.70 | 3 |
| **DB Breweries (New Zealand)** | | | | | |
| DB Draught | 12 | 09.60 | 109 | 04.00 | 2 |
| DB Bitter | 12 | 09.60 | 109 | 03.50 | 2 |
| Export Gold | 12 | 09.60 | 117 | 04.00 | 2 |
| Tui EIPA | 12 | 09.60 | 117 | 04.00 | 2 |
| Export Dry | 12 | 10.29 | 117 | 05.00 | 2 |
| Flame | 12 | 10.29 | 147 | 05.20 | 3 |
| Monteith's Pilsener | 12 | 10.29 | 138 | 05.00 | 3 |
| Monteith's Golden | 12 | 10.29 | 138 | 05.00 | 3 |
| Monteith's Celtic Red | 12 | 12.00 | 134 | 04.40 | 3 |
| Monteith's Black | 12 | 15.43 | 167 | 05.20 | 3 |
| Monteith's Original | 12 | 15.43 | 159 | 05.20 | 3 |
| Moneith's Radler | 12 | | 159 | 05.00 | 3 |
| **Deschutes** | | | | | |
| Bachelor ESB | 12 | 18.80 | 180 | 05.30 | 4 |
| Black Butte Porter | 12 | 18.85 | 192 | 05.20 | 4 |
| Buzzsaw Brown | 12 | | 170 | 04.80 | 3 |
| Cascade | 12 | 14.25 | 145 | 04.50 | 3 |
| Cider Cone Red | 12 | | 180 | 05.40 | 4 |
| Inversion IPA | 12 | | 228 | 06.80 | 4 |

|  | Oz | Carbs | Cal | Abv | Weight Watcher's POINTS® |
|---|---|---|---|---|---|
| Jubelale | 12 |  | 216 | 06.70 | 4 |
| Mirror Pond Pale Ale | 12 | 17.40 | 170 | 05.00 | 3 |
| Obsidian | 12 | 20.50 | 220 | 06.40 | 4 |
| Pine Mountain Pils | 12 |  | 154 | 05.15 | 3 |
| Quail Springs IPA | 12 | 19.40 | 200 | 05.80 | 4 |
| Twilight Ale | 12 |  | 162 | 05.00 | 3 |

### Devils Canyon

|  | Oz | Carbs | Cal | Abv | Weight Watcher's POINTS® |
|---|---|---|---|---|---|
| Deadicated Amber | 12 | 21.00 | 192 | 05.60 | 4 |
| Full Boar Scotch Ale | 12 | 24.90 | 244 | 07.50 | 5 |
| Hades Habanero | 12 | 17.30 | 178 | 05.60 | 3 |
| Lager Diabla | 12 | 17.30 | 178 | 05.60 | 3 |
| Red Devil Rye IPA | 12 | 23.10 | 237 | 07.50 | 5 |
| Silicon Blonde | 12 | 18.20 | 197 | 06.40 | 4 |

### Diamond Knot

|  | Oz | Carbs | Cal | Abv | Weight Watcher's POINTS® |
|---|---|---|---|---|---|
| Golden Ale | 12 | 14.30 | 144 | 04.50 | 3 |
| Hefe-Weizen | 12 | 17.90 | 175 | 05.30 | 3 |
| Icebreaker Barley Wine | 12 | 27.00 | 294 | 09.70 | 6 |
| Industrial Ho!Ho! | 12 | 22.80 | 230 | 07.20 | 5 |
| Industrial IPA | 12 | 21.30 | 230 | 07.50 | 5 |
| IPA | 12 | 17.25 | 177 | 05.60 | 3 |
| Lighthouse | 12 | 12.10 | 131 | 04.30 | 3 |
| Possession Porter | 12 | 17.00 | 171 | 05.30 | 3 |
| Rivertown Brown | 12 | 17.00 | 171 | 05.30 | 3 |
| Steamer Glide Stout | 12 | 14.30 | 144 | 04.50 | 3 |

### Dogfish Head

|  | Oz | Carbs | Cal | Abv | Weight Watcher's POINTS® |
|---|---|---|---|---|---|
| 60 Minute IPA | 12 |  | 209 | 06.00 | 4 |
| 90 Minute IPA | 12 |  | 294 | 09.00 | 6 |

| | Oz | Carbs | Cal | Abv | Weight Watcher's POINTS® |
|---|---|---|---|---|---|
| 120 Minute IPA | 12 | | 450 | 20.00 | 9 |
| Aprihop | 12 | | 240 | 07.00 | 5 |
| Brown Ale | 12 | | 238 | 07.20 | 5 |
| Festina | 12 | | 160 | 04.50 | 3 |
| Midas Touch | 12 | | 307 | 09.00 | 6 |
| Punkin Ale | 12 | | 230 | 07.00 | 5 |
| Raison d'Etre | 12 | | 220 | 08.00 | 4 |
| Raison d'Extra | 12 | | 425 | 18.00 | 8 |
| Shelter Pale Ale | 12 | | 168 | 05.00 | 3 |
| World Wide Stout | 12 | | 372 | 18.00 | 7 |

## Dortmunder Aktien (DAB – Germany)

| | Oz | Carbs | Cal | Abv | Weight Watcher's POINTS® |
|---|---|---|---|---|---|
| Andreas Pils | 12 | 13.30 | 149 | 04.90 | 3 |
| Diät Pils | 500 ml | 03.50 | 116 | 04.80 | 2 |
| Export | 12 | | 153 | 05.00 | 3 |
| Hansa Alt | 12 | 14.60 | 152 | 04.80 | 3 |
| Hansa Export | 12 | 15.70 | 159 | 05.00 | 3 |
| Hansa Hefeweizen | 12 | 14.20 | 152 | 04.90 | 3 |
| Hansa Malz | 12 | 39.50 | 165 | 00.00 | 3 |
| Hansa Pils | 12 | 12.80 | 145 | 04.80 | 3 |
| Pilsener | 12 | | 139 | 04.80 | 3 |
| Stades Leicht | 12 | 10.80 | 097 | 02.80 | 2 |
| Stifts Pils | 12 | 13.30 | 149 | 04.90 | 3 |
| Strong | 12 | | 135 | 04.90 | 3 |
| Thier Pils | 12 | 13.30 | 149 | 04.90 | 3 |

## Dragonmead

| | Oz | Carbs | Cal | Abv | Weight Watcher's POINTS® |
|---|---|---|---|---|---|
| 6Ts Dortmunder | 12 | 14.30 | 176 | 06.10 | 3 |
| Armageddon Grand Cru | 12 | 34.90 | 364 | 11.60 | 7 |

| | Oz | Carbs | Cal | Abv | Weight Watcher's POINTS® |
|---|---|---|---|---|---|
| Bill's Witbier | 12 | 17.50 | 165 | 04.90 | 3 |
| Bishop Bob's Holy Smoke | 12 | 14.60 | 167 | 05.60 | 3 |
| Bock Tubock | 12 | 29.50 | 262 | 07.50 | 5 |
| Broken Paddle India Pale Ale | 12 | 20.50 | 198 | 06.00 | 4 |
| Bronze Griffin Belgian Ale | 12 | 25.10 | 232 | 06.80 | 5 |
| Copper Shield Bitter Harvest | 12 | 24.70 | 287 | 09.70 | 6 |
| Corktown Red | 12 | 24.20 | 212 | 06.00 | 4 |
| Crooked Door Amber Ale | 12 | 17.10 | 165 | 05.00 | 3 |
| Crusader Dark Mild Ale | 12 | 17.80 | 156 | 04.40 | 3 |
| Dead Monk Abbey Ale | 12 | 31.90 | 283 | 08.00 | 6 |
| Dragon English Bitter | 12 | 18.80 | 163 | 04.50 | 3 |
| Dragonslayer Altbier | 12 | 17.90 | 159 | 04.50 | 3 |
| Dubbel Dragon Ale | 12 | 21.00 | 223 | 07.20 | 4 |
| Earl's Spit Stout | 12 | 25.50 | 220 | 06.20 | 4 |
| Erik the Red | 12 | 11.80 | 143 | 05.00 | 3 |
| Excalibur Barley Wine | 12 | 31.00 | 343 | 11.25 | 7 |
| Final Absolution Belgian Style Trippel | 12 | 28.90 | 281 | 08.50 | 6 |
| Guinevere's Golden Belgian Ale | 12 | 17.00 | 156 | 04.50 | 3 |
| Honey Porter | 12 | 27.60 | 200 | 04.60 | 4 |
| Imperial Stout | 12 | 30.00 | 266 | 07.50 | 5 |
| Inquisition Pale Ale | 12 | 19.50 | 176 | 05.10 | 3 |

| | Oz | Carbs | Cal | Abv | Weight Watcher's POINTS® |
|---|---|---|---|---|---|
| Jul Øl | 12 | 20.50 | 198 | 06.00 | 4 |
| Kaiser's Kölsch | 12 | 13.00 | 156 | 05.40 | 3 |
| Larry's Lionheart Pale Ale | 12 | 24.50 | 188 | 04.70 | 4 |
| London Brown Ale | 12 | 17.20 | 159 | 04.70 | 3 |
| Mariann's Honey Brown | 12 | 22.70 | 196 | 05.50 | 4 |
| Nagelweiss Wheat Beer | 12 | 14.90 | 158 | 05.10 | 3 |
| Oktoberfest Marzen | 12 | 18.70 | 191 | 06.00 | 4 |
| Rev. Fred's Oatmeal Stout | 12 | 22.10 | 199 | 05.70 | 4 |
| Sir William's Extra Special Bitter | 12 | 18.20 | 166 | 04.80 | 3 |
| Squire Pilsen | 12 | 17.90 | 159 | 04.50 | 3 |
| Tafelbier Lager | 12 | 14.40 | 179 | 06.30 | 3 |
| Tayken Abock | 12 | 26.90 | 242 | 07.00 | 5 |
| Tuhelles Enbock | 12 | 22.20 | 218 | 06.70 | 4 |
| Under the Kilt Wee Heavy | 12 | 28.50 | 265 | 07.80 | 5 |
| Woody's Perfect Porter | 12 | 20.40 | 164 | 04.30 | 3 |

## Dry Dock

| | Oz | Carbs | Cal | Abv | Weight Watcher's POINTS® |
|---|---|---|---|---|---|
| Apricot Blonde | 12 | 24.50 | 188 | 04.70 | 4 |
| HMS Bounty Old Ale | 12 | 31.20 | 267 | 07.30 | 5 |
| HMS Victory ESB | 12 | 24.50 | 188 | 04.70 | 4 |
| Lucky Scotsman | 12 | 15.60 | 127 | 03.30 | 2 |
| Urca Vanilla Porter | 12 | 24.40 | 200 | 05.30 | 4 |
| USS Stout | 12 | 32.10 | 258 | 06.70 | 5 |

| | Oz | Carbs | Cal | Abv | Weight Watcher's POINTS® |
|---|---|---|---|---|---|
| **Durango** | | | | | |
| Amber Ale | 12 | 15.30 | 167 | 05.50 | 3 |
| Blueberry Wheat | 12 | 15.20 | 164 | 05.30 | 3 |
| Colorfest | 12 | 18.50 | 194 | 06.20 | 4 |
| Dark Lager | 12 | 17.50 | 181 | 05.80 | 4 |
| Derail Ale | 12 | 22.40 | 254 | 08.50 | 5 |
| Golden Ale | 12 | 17.50 | 181 | 05.80 | 4 |
| Pale Ale | 12 | 17.00 | 186 | 06.10 | 4 |
| Wheat Beer | 12 | 15.20 | 164 | 05.30 | 3 |
| Winter Ale | 12 | 19.00 | 198 | 06.30 | 4 |
| **Empyrean** | | | | | |
| Better World Belgian-Style Wheat | 12 | 17.70 | 155 | 04.30 | 3 |
| Burning Skye Scottish Style Ale | 12 | 15.30 | 173 | 05.80 | 3 |
| Chaco Canyon Honey Gold | 12 | 16.90 | 161 | 04.80 | 3 |
| Collapsar Oatmeal Stout | 12 | 21.00 | 200 | 06.00 | 4 |
| Dark Side Vanilla Porter | 12 | 21.10 | 196 | 05.70 | 4 |
| Fallen Angel Sweet Stout | 12 | 19.00 | 182 | 05.50 | 4 |
| LunaSea ESB | 12 | 17.70 | 193 | 06.30 | 4 |
| Third Stone Brown | 12 | 19.80 | 182 | 05.30 | 4 |
| Martian Alt-er Ego FallFest | 12 | 18.10 | 178 | 05.50 | 3 |
| Super Nova Summer Common Beer | 12 | 17.80 | 187 | 06.00 | 4 |

|  | Oz | Carbs | Cal | Abv | Weight Watcher's POINTS® |
|---|---|---|---|---|---|

### Erdinger (Germany)

|  | Oz | Carbs | Cal | Abv | Pts |
|---|---|---|---|---|---|
| Alkoholfrei | 12 | 18.71 | 089 | 00.40 | 2 |
| Champ | 12 | 15.40 | 150 | 04.70 | 3 |
| Dunkel | 12 | 15.50 | 170 | 05.60 | 3 |
| Kristall | 12 | 15.20 | 160 | 05.30 | 3 |
| Leicht | 12 | 11.50 | 100 | 02.90 | 2 |
| Pikantus | 12 | 21.70 | 225 | 07.30 | 4 |
| Schneeweisse | 12 | 15.50 | 170 | 05.60 | 3 |
| Urweisse | 12 | 16.90 | 165 | 05.20 | 3 |
| Weissbier | 12 | 15.20 | 160 | 05.30 | 3 |

### Faust (Germany)

|  | Oz | Carbs | Cal | Abv | Pts |
|---|---|---|---|---|---|
| Doppelbock | 12 | 31.70 | 263 | 07.00 | 5 |
| Export | 12 | 17.00 | 170 | 05.30 | 3 |
| Festbier | 12 | 17.80 | 178 | 05.50 | 3 |
| Hefe-Weizen Dunkel | 12 | 16.40 | 166 | 05.20 | 3 |
| Hefe-Weizen Hell | 12 | 16.30 | 165 | 05.10 | 3 |
| Kräusen | 12 | 17.90 | 179 | 05.50 | 3 |
| Leicht | 12 | 10.20 | 097 | 02.60 | 2 |
| Pils | 12 | 15.60 | 160 | 04.90 | 3 |
| Winterfestbier | 12 | 17.90 | 179 | 05.50 | 3 |

### Fearless

|  | Oz | Carbs | Cal | Abv | Pts |
|---|---|---|---|---|---|
| Bennett's Pale Ale | 12 | 20.40 | 180 | 05.10 | 4 |
| Cream Ale | 12 | 10.90 | 137 | 04.80 | 3 |
| IPA | 12 | 17.10 | 165 | 05.00 | 3 |
| Maibock | 12 | 23.40 | 243 | 07.70 | 5 |
| Porter | 12 | 20.80 | 180 | 05.00 | 4 |
| Scottish Ale | 12 | 17.90 | 175 | 05.30 | 3 |
| Strong Scotch Ale | 12 | 27.40 | 264 | 08.00 | 5 |

|  | Oz | Carbs | Cal | Abv | Weight Watcher's POINTS® |
|---|---|---|---|---|---|
| Tomahawk Brown | 12 | 17.90 | 175 | 05.30 | 3 |

## FEMSA (Mexico)

|  | Oz | Carbs | Cal | Abv | POINTS |
|---|---|---|---|---|---|
| Dos Equis Amber | 12 | 12.87 | 145 | 04.80 | 3 |
| Tecate | 12 | 12.50 | 142 | 04.30 | 3 |

## Firehouse

|  | Oz | Carbs | Cal | Abv | POINTS |
|---|---|---|---|---|---|
| Hefeweizen | 12 | 15.70 | 160 | 05.00 | 3 |
| Pale Ale | 12 | 16.60 | 179 | 05.80 | 3 |
| Porter | 12 | 16.10 | 168 | 05.30 | 3 |
| Red Ale | 12 | 17.00 | 187 | 06.10 | 4 |

## Fish

|  | Oz | Carbs | Cal | Abv | POINTS |
|---|---|---|---|---|---|
| Dentonator Doppelbock | 12 | 27.40 | 274 | 08.50 | 5 |
| Dunkel Weizen | 12 | 27.30 | 199 | 04.70 | 4 |
| Friesian Pilsener | 12 | 34.30 | 222 | 04.40 | 4 |
| Hodgson's IPA | 12 | 25.00 | 207 | 05.50 | 4 |
| Ingalls ESB | 12 | 22.70 | 197 | 05.50 | 4 |
| Leviathan Barleywine | 12 | 31.40 | 319 | 10.00 | 6 |
| Mudshark Porter | 12 | 21.70 | 199 | 05.80 | 4 |
| Oktoberfest | 12 | 28.20 | 219 | 05.50 | 4 |
| Organic IPA | 12 | 17.50 | 196 | 06.50 | 4 |
| Organic Pale Ale | 12 | 19.90 | 186 | 05.50 | 4 |
| Poseiden's Imperial Stout | 12 | 42.00 | 338 | 08.80 | 7 |
| Thorton Creek Pale Ale | 12 | 22.60 | 187 | 05.00 | 4 |
| Trout Stout | 12 | 21.80 | 193 | 05.50 | 4 |
| Wild Salmon Organic Pale Ale | 12 | 12.60 | 156 | 05.50 | 3 |
| Winterfish Pale Ale | 12 | 25.80 | 239 | 07.00 | 5 |

| | Oz | Carbs | Cal | Abv | Weight Watcher's POINTS® |
|---|---|---|---|---|---|
| Whistling Pig | 12 | 19.00 | 182 | 05.50 | 4 |

### Fitger's

| | | | | | |
|---|---|---|---|---|---|
| El Nino Double Hopped IPA | 12 | 18.70 | 222 | 07.60 | 4 |
| Mariner Mild | 12 | 13.75 | 119 | 03.30 | 2 |
| Starfile Pale | 12 | 15.20 | 195 | 06.90 | 4 |
| Farmhouse | 12 | 14.40 | 210 | 07.40 | 4 |
| Sterling Select | 12 | 14.60 | 182 | 06.40 | 4 |
| Apricot Wheat | 12 | 11.20 | 159 | 05.50 | 3 |

### Flat Branch

| | | | | | |
|---|---|---|---|---|---|
| Brown | 12 | 23.70 | 188 | 04.80 | 4 |
| Green Chili | 12 | 17.45 | 165 | 04.90 | 3 |
| Honey Wheat | 12 | 19.75 | 182 | 05.30 | 4 |
| Hudson ESB | 12 | 24.30 | 231 | 06.90 | 5 |
| IPA | 12 | 22.15 | 199 | 05.70 | 4 |
| Katy Trail Pale Ale | 12 | 18.60 | 175 | 05.20 | 3 |
| Lager | 12 | 19.05 | 185 | 05.60 | 4 |
| Oil Change Stout | 12 | 22.80 | 198 | 05.60 | 4 |

### Flying Dog

| | | | | | |
|---|---|---|---|---|---|
| Classic Pale Ale | 12 | 11.40 | 146 | 05.50 | 3 |
| Dogtoberfest | 12 | 11.40 | 158 | 05.30 | 3 |
| Double Dog | 12 | 15.00 | 292 | 11.50 | 6 |
| Garde Dog | 12 | 11.40 | 158 | 05.50 | 3 |
| Gonzo Imperial | 12 | 18.60 | 269 | 07.80 | 5 |
| Horn Dog | 12 | 18.90 | 314 | 10.20 | 6 |
| In-Heat Wheat | 12 | 08.30 | 131 | 04.70 | 3 |
| K-9 Cruiser | 12 | 10.60 | 181 | 06.40 | 4 |
| Kerberos Tripel | 12 | 18.60 | 269 | 08.50 | 5 |

| | Oz | Carbs | Cal | Abv | Weight Watcher's POINTS® |
|---|---|---|---|---|---|
| Old Scratch | 12 | 09.60 | 150 | 05.50 | 3 |
| Road Dog | 12 | 12.00 | 158 | 06.00 | 3 |
| Snake Dog | 12 | 10.60 | 179 | 07.10 | 3 |
| Trite Bite | 12 | 07.10 | 124 | 05.00 | 2 |
| Woody Creek | 12 | 08.30 | 131 | 04.80 | 3 |

## Flying Fish

| | Oz | Carbs | Cal | Abv | |
|---|---|---|---|---|---|
| Porter | 12 | 19.00 | 182 | 05.60 | 4 |
| Belgian Ale Double | 12 | 15.75 | 208 | 07.00 | 4 |
| ESB | 12 | 19.90 | 185 | 05.50 | 4 |
| Extra Pale Ale | 12 | 14.40 | 148 | 04.80 | 3 |

## Foster's (Australia)

| | Oz | Carbs | Cal | Abv | |
|---|---|---|---|---|---|
| Abbotsford Invalid Stout | 12 | 11.72 | 160 | 05.20 | 3 |
| Beez Neez | 12 | 11.36 | 142 | 04.70 | 3 |
| Bohemian Pilzner | 12 | 14.56 | 153 | 04.70 | 3 |
| Carlton Black Ale | 12 | 10.65 | 131 | 04.40 | 3 |
| Carlton Cold Filtered Bitter | 12 | 09.59 | 131 | 04.60 | 3 |
| Carlton Cold Ultra Chill | 12 | 10.30 | 170 | 06.50 | 3 |
| Carlton Draught | 12 | 09.59 | 131 | 04.60 | 3 |
| Carlton Dry Fusion | 12 | 07.81 | 117 | 04.20 | 2 |
| Carlton Empire | 12 | 09.94 | 135 | 04.60 | 3 |
| Carlton Light | 12 | 10.65 | 096 | 02.70 | 2 |
| Carlton LJ | 12 | 03.20 | 107 | 04.60 | 2 |
| Carlton Mid Strength Bitter | 12 | 14.20 | 128 | 03.50 | 2 |
| Carlton Dry | 12 | 09.94 | 131 | 04.50 | 3 |
| Carlton Sterling | 12 | 11.00 | 096 | 02.50 | 2 |

| | Oz | Carbs | Cal | Abv | Weight Watcher's POINTS® |
|---|---|---|---|---|---|
| Cascade Amber Ale | 12 | 15.27 | 160 | 04.80 | 3 |
| Cascade Autumn Amber | 12 | 15.98 | 167 | 05.00 | 3 |
| Cascade Bitter | 12 | 09.59 | 124 | 04.40 | 2 |
| Cascade Blonde Lager | 12 | 12.43 | 146 | 04.80 | 3 |
| Cascade Draught | 12 | 09.23 | 135 | 04.70 | 3 |
| Cascade First Harvest | 12 | 14.20 | 170 | 05.50 | 3 |
| Cascade Green | 12 | 05.65 | 114 | 04.50 | 2 |
| Cascade Lager | 12 | 09.59 | 138 | 04.80 | 3 |
| Cascade Pale Ale | 12 | 09.94 | 146 | 05.00 | 3 |
| Cascade Premium | 12 | 11.00 | 149 | 05.20 | 3 |
| Cascade Premium Light | 12 | 11.36 | 103 | 02.80 | 2 |
| Cascade Spring Fest | 12 | 12.78 | 153 | 05.00 | 3 |
| Cascade Stout | 12 | 15.98 | 181 | 05.80 | 4 |
| Cascade Summer Blonde | 12 | 13.14 | 153 | 05.00 | 3 |
| Cascade Winter Warmer | 12 | 14.91 | 163 | 05.20 | 3 |
| Crown Gold | 12 | 11.00 | 117 | 03.50 | 2 |
| Crown Lager | 12 | 11.00 | 142 | 04.90 | 3 |
| Fiji Bitter | 12 | 09.94 | 135 | 04.60 | 3 |
| Fiji Gold | 12 | 05.68 | 117 | 04.60 | 2 |
| Foster's Lager | 12 | 11.00 | 142 | 04.90 | 3 |
| Foster's Light-NZ | 12 | 10.30 | 107 | 02.50 | 2 |
| Foster's Light Ice | 12 | 13.49 | 099 | 02.30 | 2 |
| Foster's Special Bitter | 12 | 12.78 | 103 | 02.50 | 3 |

|  | Oz | Carbs | Cal | Abv | Weight Watcher's POINTS® |
|---|---|---|---|---|---|
| Guinness Draught | 12 | 12.78 | 138 | 04.20 | 3 |
| Guinness | 12 | 17.40 | 192 | 06.00 | 4 |
| 303 Ice Gold | 12 | 11.76 | 114 | 03.30 | 2 |
| KB Lager | 12 | 11.00 | 131 | 04.40 | 3 |
| Kent Old Brown | 12 | 11.36 | 135 | 04.40 | 3 |
| Matilda Bay Premium Lager | 12 | 13.85 | 124 | 03.40 | 2 |
| Melbourne Bitter | 12 | 11.00 | 142 | 04.90 | 3 |
| NT Draught | 12 | 09.94 | 138 | 04.90 | 3 |
| Power's Bitter | 12 | 09.94 | 128 | 04.40 | 2 |
| Power's Gold | 12 | 09.23 | 103 | 03.20 | 2 |
| Power's Ice | 12 | 08.88 | 128 | 04.50 | 2 |
| Pure Blond | 12 | 03.20 | 107 | 04.60 | 2 |
| Redback Cristal | 12 | 12.43 | 142 | 04.50 | 3 |
| Redback Mild | 12 | 09.59 | 110 | 03.40 | 2 |
| Redback Original | 12 | 12.78 | 146 | 04.70 | 3 |
| Resch's DA | 12 | 11.76 | 135 | 04.40 | 3 |
| Resch's Draught | 12 | 09.94 | 131 | 04.50 | 3 |
| Resch's Pilsener | 12 | 10.30 | 131 | 04.40 | 3 |
| Resch's Pils (NZ) | 12 | 08.88 | 117 | 04.00 | 2 |
| Resch's Real Bitter | 12 | 10.65 | 128 | 04.00 | 2 |
| Resch's Real Bitter (NZ) | 12 | 10.65 | 124 | 04.00 | 2 |
| Richmond Lager | 12 | 09.94 | 138 | 04.90 | 3 |
| Sheaf Stout | 12 | 18.82 | 188 | 05.70 | 4 |
| Stella Artois | 12 | 12.78 | 153 | 05.10 | 3 |
| Victoria Bitter | 12 | 11.00 | 142 | 04.90 | 3 |
| Victoria Bitter Mid-Strength | 12 | 10.30 | 114 | 03.50 | 2 |

|  | Oz | Carbs | Cal | Abv | Weight Watcher's POINTS® |
|---|---|---|---|---|---|
| Victoria Bitter Org Ale | 12 | 13.49 | 149 | 04.60 | 3 |
| WA Gold | 12 | 11.72 | 110 | 03.00 | 2 |
| Yatala Pilsen | 12 | 10.30 | 138 | 04.80 | 3 |

### Franziskaner (Germany)

|  | Oz | Carbs | Cal | Abv | Weight Watcher's POINTS® |
|---|---|---|---|---|---|
| Hefe-Weissbier | 12 | 09.59 | 153 | 05.00 | 3 |
| Hefe-Weissbier Dunkel | 12 | 09.86 | 156 | 05.00 | 3 |
| Hefe-Weissbier Kristallklar | 12 | 09.59 | 153 | 05.00 | 3 |

### Fuller Smith (UK)

|  | Oz | Carbs | Cal | Abv | Weight Watcher's POINTS® |
|---|---|---|---|---|---|
| Summer Ale | 12 | 12.00 | 124 | 04.00 | 2 |

### Full Sail

|  | Oz | Carbs | Cal | Abv | Weight Watcher's POINTS® |
|---|---|---|---|---|---|
| Amber | 12 | 17.00 | 175 | 05.50 | 3 |
| IPA | 12 | 17.00 | 186 | 06.00 | 4 |
| LTD 01 | 12 | 18.00 | 205 | 06.40 | 4 |
| LTD 02 | 12 | 18.00 | 205 | 06.40 | 4 |
| Pale Ale | 12 | 16.00 | 172 | 05.40 | 3 |
| Session | 12 | 12.50 | 140 | 05.10 | 3 |
| Wassail | 12 | 19.40 | 220 | 07.00 | 4 |

### Furthermore

|  | Oz | Carbs | Cal | Abv | Weight Watcher's POINTS® |
|---|---|---|---|---|---|
| Knot Stock | 12 | 24.30 | 204 | 05.50 | 4 |
| Oscura | 12 | 25.70 | 205 | 05.30 | 4 |
| Proper | 12 | 18.60 | 162 | 04.50 | 3 |
| Three-Feet Stout | 12 | 22.70 | 197 | 05.50 | 4 |

### Fustlich Ferstenbergische (Germany)

|  | Oz | Carbs | Cal | Abv | Weight Watcher's POINTS® |
|---|---|---|---|---|---|
| Fürstenberg | 12 |  | 138 | 04.40 | 3 |

|  | Oz | Carbs | Cal | Abv | Weight Watcher's POINTS® |
|---|---|---|---|---|---|
| **Garrison (Canada)** | | | | | |
| Grand Baltic Porter | 12 | 27.10 | 283 | 09.00 | 6 |
| Imperial Pale Ale | 12 | 24.30 | 232 | 06.90 | 5 |
| Irish Red | 12 | 17.10 | 165 | 05.00 | 3 |
| Martello Stout | 12 | 21.20 | 174 | 04.60 | 3 |
| Nut Brown Ale | 12 | 18.90 | 173 | 05.00 | 3 |
| Raspberry Wheat | 12 | 13.90 | 145 | 04.60 | 3 |
| Tall Ship Amber | 12 | 14.80 | 148 | 04.60 | 3 |
| Winter Warmer | 12 | 20.40 | 211 | 06.70 | 4 |
| **Gentle Ben's** | | | | | |
| Amber | 12 | 15.50 | 170 | 05.60 | 3 |
| Blonde | 12 | 12.40 | 138 | 04.50 | 3 |
| Hefeweizen | 12 | 18.70 | 222 | 07.60 | 4 |
| IPA | 12 | 18.70 | 222 | 07.60 | 4 |
| Nut Brown | 12 | 15.20 | 164 | 05.30 | 3 |
| Oatmeal Stout | 12 | 21.40 | 193 | 05.50 | 4 |
| Pale Ale | 12 | 15.20 | 164 | 05.30 | 3 |
| Porter | 12 | 21.00 | 192 | 05.60 | 4 |
| **Georgetown** | | | | | |
| Pale Ale | 12 | 15.90 | 171 | 05.50 | 3 |
| Pilsner | 12 | 15.60 | 158 | 04.90 | 3 |
| Red Ale | 12 | 21.10 | 211 | 06.50 | 4 |
| **Gordon Biersch** | | | | | |
| Blonde Bock | 12 | 15.81 | 208 | 07.10 | 4 |
| Hefeweizen | 12 | | 164 | 05.50 | 3 |
| Märzen | 12 | | 174 | 05.60 | 3 |
| Pilsner | 12 | | 154 | 05.30 | 3 |
| Winter Bock | 12 | | 234 | 07.50 | 5 |

|  | Oz | Carbs | Cal | Abv | Weight Watcher's POINTS® |
|---|---|---|---|---|---|
| **Goose Island** | | | | | |
| American Wheat "312" | 12 | 10.50 | 130 | 04.36 | 3 |
| Blonde Ale | 12 | 12.70 | 143 | 04.80 | 3 |
| Bourbon County Stout | 12 | 45.00 | 415 | 13.50 | 8 |
| Christmas Ale | 12 | 30.00 | 240 | 05.50 | 5 |
| Demolition | 12 | 24.00 | 245 | 06.70 | 5 |
| Harvest Ale | 12 | 20.00 | 200 | 05.70 | 4 |
| Hex Nut Brown | 12 | 16.50 | 171 | 05.00 | 3 |
| Honker's Ale | 12 | 16.50 | 150 | 04.30 | 3 |
| Imperial Brown Goose | 12 | 30.00 | 255 | 08.20 | 5 |
| Imperial IPA | 12 | 30.00 | 255 | 09.00 | 5 |
| India Pale Ale | 12 | 23.50 | 200 | 05.90 | 4 |
| Juliet | 12 | 17.00 | 192 | 06.70 | 4 |
| Kilgubbin Irish Red Ale | 12 | 15.00 | 160 | 04.50 | 3 |
| Lamar St Pale Ale | 12 | 15.00 | 160 | 04.30 | 3 |
| Matilda | 12 | 18.00 | 195 | 07.00 | 4 |
| Mild Winter | 12 | 22.00 | 220 | 05.60 | 4 |
| Nut Brown Ale | 12 | 17.50 | 200 | 05.30 | 4 |
| Oatmeal Stout | 12 | 24.00 | 160 | 05.10 | 3 |
| Oktoberfest Lager | 12 | 17.00 | 180 | 05.40 | 4 |
| Pere Jacques | 12 | 30.00 | 300 | 07.80 | 6 |
| Pils Lager | 12 | 13.00 | 155 | 04.90 | 3 |
| Summertime Kolsch | 12 | 13.50 | 150 | 04.70 | 3 |

|  | Oz | Carbs | Cal | Abv | Weight Watcher's POINTS® |
|---|---|---|---|---|---|
| **Grand Teton** | | | | | |
| Bitch Creek | 12 | 25.20 | 207 | 05.50 | 4 |
| Old Faithful Ale | 12 | 19.90 | 175 | 04.95 | 3 |
| Organic Blond Ale | 12 | 19.30 | 173 | 04.95 | 3 |
| Sweetgrass IPA | 12 | 25.20 | 207 | 05.50 | 4 |
| Teton Ale | 12 | 21.10 | 180 | 04.98 | 4 |
| Workhorse Wheat | 12 | 15.50 | 140 | 04.00 | 3 |
| **Granite (Canada)** | | | | | |
| Best Bitter | 12 | 16.10 | 152 | 04.50 | 3 |
| Best Bitter Special | 12 | 16.10 | 152 | 04.50 | 3 |
| IPA | 12 | 15.50 | 170 | 05.20 | 3 |
| Keefe's Irish Stout | 12 | 17.90 | 159 | 04.50 | 3 |
| Peculiar | 12 | 19.20 | 185 | 05.60 | 4 |
| Ringberry | 12 | 17.00 | 171 | 05.30 | 3 |
| Ringwood | 12 | 17.00 | 171 | 05.30 | 3 |
| Summer Ale | 12 | 14.00 | 138 | 04.30 | 3 |
| **Great Divide** | | | | | |
| Arapahoe Amber | 12 | 18.85 | 179 | 05.30 | 3 |
| Bee Sting | 12 | 15.70 | 174 | 05.70 | 3 |
| Denver Pale Ale | 12 | 16.20 | 171 | 05.50 | 3 |
| Fresh Hop | 12 | 18.20 | 197 | 06.40 | 4 |
| Hercules Double IPA | 12 | 28.80 | 296 | 09.30 | 6 |
| Hibernation | 12 | 26.50 | 264 | 08.10 | 5 |
| St. Brigid's Porter | 12 | 17.60 | 184 | 05.90 | 4 |
| Titan IPA | 12 | 21.00 | 223 | 07.20 | 4 |
| Wild Raspberry Ale | 12 | 15.45 | 170 | 05.60 | 3 |
| Yeti Imperial Stout | 12 | 32.60 | 329 | 10.30 | 6 |

|  | Oz | Carbs | Cal | Abv | Weight Watcher's POINTS® |
|---|---|---|---|---|---|
| **Great Waters** | | | | | |
| Black Watch Oat Stout | 12 | 23.10 | 204 | 05.80 | 4 |
| Brew # 700 | 12 | 28.30 | 237 | 06.40 | 5 |
| Brown Trout Brown Ale | 12 | 23.00 | 204 | 05.80 | 4 |
| Golden Prairie Blond Ale | 12 | 13.70 | 148 | 04.80 | 3 |
| Great Waters House Ale | 12 | 15.80 | 160 | 05.00 | 3 |
| Mr. Smooth Dark Mild | 12 | 08.90 | 132 | 05.00 | 3 |
| Pflugenpflagen | 12 | 23.10 | 222 | 06.70 | 4 |
| Saint Peter Pale Ale | 12 | 20.80 | 181 | 05.50 | 4 |
| **Green Bamboo (China)** | | | | | |
| Great Wall | 12 | | 160 | 04.60 | 3 |
| **Greenall Whitley (UK)** | | | | | |
| Cheshire English Pub Beer | 12 | | 142 | 05.00 | 3 |
| Chester Golden Ale | 12 | | 156 | 05.40 | 3 |
| **Grolsch (Holland)** | | | | | |
| Amber | 12 | 11.36 | 153 | 03.90 | 3 |
| Herfstbok | 12 | 15.62 | 204 | 05.40 | 4 |
| Oud Bruin | 12 | 12.78 | 112 | 01.80 | 2 |
| Premium Pilsner | 12 | 11.00 | 149 | 04.00 | 3 |
| Special Malt | 12 | 18.46 | 072 | 00.04 | 1 |
| Wintarvorst | 12 | 17.40 | 217 | 07.00 | 4 |
| Zomergoud | 12 | 11.36 | 153 | 05.00 | 3 |
| **Grupo Modelo (Mexico)** | | | | | |
| Corona Extra | 12 | 13.99 | 148 | 04.60 | 3 |
| Corona Light | 12 | 05.00 | 105 | 03.70 | 2 |

|  | Oz | Carbs | Cal | Abv | Weight Watcher's POINTS® |
|---|---|---|---|---|---|
| Modelo Especial | 12 | 04.00 | 145 | 06.00 | 3 |
| Negra Modelo | 12 | 14.00 | 169 | 05.40 | 3 |
| Pacifico Clara | 12 | 13.00 | 146 | 04.40 | 3 |

## Guinness

Please read the Preface about Guinness and the reasons for their often inconsistent nutritional values in different countries.

|  | Oz | Carbs | Cal | Abv | Weight Watcher's POINTS® |
|---|---|---|---|---|---|
| Guinness Draught | 12 | 10.00 | 125 | 04.00 | 2 |
| Guinness Extra Stout | 12 | 14.00 | 176 | 07.50 | 3 |
| Harp Lager | 12 | 13.00 | 153 | 05.00 | 3 |
| Kaliber | 12 | 10.30 | 070 | 00.50 | 1 |

## Harpoon

|  | Oz | Carbs | Cal | Abv | Weight Watcher's POINTS® |
|---|---|---|---|---|---|
| IPA | 12 | ~15.0 | ~170 | 05.90 | 3 |

## Heineken (Holland)

|  | Oz | Carbs | Cal | Abv | Weight Watcher's POINTS® |
|---|---|---|---|---|---|
| Eindejaars Bier | 12 | 19.53 | 213 | 06.50 | 4 |
| Heineken | 12 | 10.65 | 142 | 05.00 | 3 |
| Heineken Oud Bruin | 12 | 19.70 | 124 | 02.50 | 2 |
| Heineken Tarwebok | 12 | 23.08 | 231 | 06.50 | 5 |
| Kylian | 12 | 23.08 | 231 | 06.50 | 5 |
| Lingen's Blond | 12 | 17.75 | 124 | 02.00 | 2 |
| Vollenhoven's Stout | 12 | 19.53 | 213 | 06.60 | 4 |
| Vos | 12 | 14.20 | 160 | 05.00 | 3 |
| Wieckse Witte | 12 | 12.43 | 160 | 05.00 | 3 |

## High Falls

|  | Oz | Carbs | Cal | Abv | Weight Watcher's POINTS® |
|---|---|---|---|---|---|
| Genesee Beer | 12 | 13.50 | 148 | 04.50 | 3 |
| Genesee Cream Ale | 12 | 15.00 | 162 | 05.10 | 3 |
| Genesee Ice | 12 | 14.50 | 156 | 05.90 | 3 |
| Genny Light | 12 | 05.50 | 096 | 03.60 | 2 |
| Genesee NA | 12 | 15.00 | 070 | 00.05 | 1 |
| Genesee Red | 12 | 14.00 | 148 | 04.90 | 3 |

|  | Oz | Carbs | Cal | Abv | Weight Watcher's POINTS® |
|---|---|---|---|---|---|
| JW Dundee American Amber | 12 | 13.30 | 150 | 04.90 | 3 |
| JW Dundee American Pale Ale | 12 | 13.50 | 165 | 05.30 | 3 |
| Honey Brown Lager | 12 | 13.50 | 150 | 04.50 | 3 |
| Michael Shea's Irish Amber | 12 | 13.00 | 145 | 04.62 | 3 |
| **Highland Brewing** | | | | | |
| Black Mocha Stout | 12 | 24.99 | 217 | 05.30 | 4 |
| Gaelic Ale | 12 | 17.86 | 173 | 05.80 | 3 |
| Kashmir IPA | 12 | 16.82 | 191 | 05.60 | 4 |
| Oatmeal Porter | 12 | 19.42 | 191 | 05.80 | 4 |
| St. Terese's Pale Ale | 12 | 15.65 | 170 | 05.20 | 3 |
| **Hoegaarden (Belgium)** | | | | | |
| Witbier | 12 | 13.49 | 160 | 04.90 | 3 |
| **Hopback (UK)** | | | | | |
| Summer Lightning | 12 | 11.60 | 143 | 05.00 | 3 |
| **Hopworks Urban (Organic)** | | | | | |
| Deluxe Ale | 12 | 23.40 | 228 | 06.90 | 4 |
| ESB | 12 | 20.50 | 182 | 05.20 | 4 |
| HUB Lager | 12 | 13.10 | 151 | 05.10 | 3 |
| IPA | 12 | 18.00 | 200 | 06.60 | 4 |
| Pale Ale | 12 | 15.60 | 166 | 05.30 | 3 |
| Stout | 12 | 25.30 | 205 | 05.30 | 4 |
| **Hövels (Germany)** | | | | | |
| Bitterbier | 12 | | 163 | 05.50 | 3 |
| **Ice Harbor** | | | | | |
| ESB | 12 | 21.20 | 205 | 06.20 | 4 |
| Hefeweizen | 12 | 16.40 | 159 | 04.80 | 3 |

|  | Oz | Carbs | Cal | Abv | Weight Watcher's POINTS® |
|---|---|---|---|---|---|
| IPA | 12 | 24.80 | 241 | 07.30 | 5 |
| IWA | 12 | 28.20 | 259 | 07.50 | 5 |
| Irish Stout (Nitro) | 12 | 18.80 | 148 | 03.70 | 3 |
| Nut Brown | 12 | 17.80 | 172 | 05.20 | 3 |
| Pale Ale | 12 | 20.50 | 204 | 06.30 | 4 |
| Pilsner | 12 | 23.30 | 225 | 06.80 | 4 |
| Red Ale | 12 | 12.90 | 163 | 05.70 | 4 |
| Scottish Ale | 12 | 17.90 | 159 | 04.50 | 3 |
| Stout | 12 | 16.80 | 174 | 05.50 | 3 |
| Summer Lager | 12 | 13.90 | 157 | 05.20 | 3 |
| Wallula Red | 12 | 22.10 | 215 | 06.50 | 4 |

### Independence

|  | Oz | Carbs | Cal | Abv | Weight Watcher's POINTS® |
|---|---|---|---|---|---|
| Amber | 12 | 13.80 | 145 | 04.90 | 3 |
| Bootlegger Brown | 12 | 19.60 | 195 | 06.00 | 4 |
| Freestyle | 12 | 14.40 | 144 | 4.70 | 3 |
| Independence Pale Ale | 12 | 18.20 | 178 | 05.50 | 3 |
| Jasperilla | 12 | 17.90 | 252 | 09.30 | 5 |
| Kolsch | 12 | 11.20 | 146 | 05.20 | 3 |
| OMA | 12 | 23.00 | 202 | 05.70 | 4 |
| Red Ale | 12 | 16.90 | 186 | 06.10 | 4 |

### Iron City

|  | Oz | Carbs | Cal | Abv | Weight Watcher's POINTS® |
|---|---|---|---|---|---|
| Augustiner | 12 | 10.00 | 135 | 04.30 | 3 |
| Iron City Beer | 12 | 10.00 | 140 | 04.50 | 3 |
| Iron City Light | 12 | 02.80 | 095 | 04.15 | 2 |

### Jacobsen (Denmark)

|  | Oz | Carbs | Cal | Abv | Weight Watcher's POINTS® |
|---|---|---|---|---|---|
| Branley Wit | 12 | 09.94 | 149 | 04.60 | 3 |
| Extra Pils | 12 | 16.33 | 192 | 05.50 | 4 |

| | Oz | Carbs | Cal | Abv | Weight Watcher's POINTS® |
|---|---|---|---|---|---|
| Golden Naked Christmas Ale | 12 | 19.17 | 245 | 07.50 | 5 |
| Original Dark Lager | 12 | 16.69 | 192 | 05.80 | 4 |
| **Käki (Finland)** | | | | | |
| Juniper Flavored | 12 | 12.78 | 153 | 04.50 | 3 |
| **Kalamazoo (Bell's)** | | | | | |
| Amber Ale | 12 | 18.00 | 190 | 06.00 | 4 |
| Best Brown Ale | 12 | 20.00 | 192 | 05.80 | 4 |
| Cherry Stout | 12 | 34.50 | 275 | 08.50 | 5 |
| Consecrator Doppelbock | 12 | 28.25 | 280 | 08.00 | 6 |
| Expedition Stout | 12 | 34.70 | 400 | 10.05 | 8 |
| Hell Hath No Fury | 12 | 36.00 | 295 | 07.70 | 6 |
| Hopslam Ale | 12 | 23.00 | 280 | 10.00 | 6 |
| Java Stout | 12 | 25.00 | 255 | 07.50 | 5 |
| Kalamazoo Stout | 12 | 23.22 | 220 | 06.00 | 4 |
| Lager | 12 | 17.00 | 170 | 05.00 | 3 |
| Oberon Ale | 12 | 17.75 | 190 | 05.80 | 4 |
| Octoberfest | 12 | 19.80 | 182 | 05.50 | 4 |
| Pale Ale | 12 | 14.20 | 165 | 05.20 | 3 |
| Porter | 12 | 15.90 | 190 | 05.60 | 4 |
| Sparkling Ale | 12 | 17.00 | 270 | 09.00 | 5 |
| Special Double Cream Stout | 12 | 25.00 | 240 | 06.10 | 5 |
| Third Coast Beer | 12 | 17.00 | 150 | 04.80 | 3 |
| Third Coast Old Ale | 12 | 14.10 | 335 | 10.20 | 7 |
| Two Hearted Ale | 12 | 12.70 | 210 | 07.00 | 4 |
| Winter White Ale | 12 | 19.20 | 171 | 05.00 | 3 |

|  | Oz | Carbs | Cal | Abv | Weight Watcher's POINTS® |
|---|---|---|---|---|---|
| **Karhupanimo (Finland)** | | | | | |
| Kirjurin Vaalea | 12 | 10.65 | 142 | 04.50 | 3 |
| Jouluolut | 12 | 18.11 | 213 | 06.50 | 4 |
| Mustakarhu | 12 | 12.78 | 160 | 05.00 | 3 |
| Oktoberfest | 12 | 14.20 | 178 | 05.20 | 3 |
| **Kennebunkport/Shipyard** | | | | | |
| Shipyard Light | 12 | 07.40 | 097 | 03.20 | 2 |
| **Kilkenny (Ireland)** | | | | | |
| Irish Beer | 12 | 10.65 | 131 | 04.30 | 3 |
| **Kirin (Japan)** | | | | | |
| Ichiban | 12 | 11.23 | 145 | 04.95 | 3 |
| Light | 12 | 08.00 | 095 | 03.31 | 3 |
| **Kiuchi (Japan)** | | | | | |
| Japanese Classic Ale | 12 | 29.40 | 253 | 07.00 | 5 |
| Pale Ale | 12 | 20.80 | 180 | 05.00 | 4 |
| Red Rice Ale | 12 | 24.00 | 231 | 07.00 | 5 |
| Sweet Stout | 11.2 | 22.10 | 162 | 03.80 | 3 |
| Weizen | 11.2 | 20.80 | 180 | 05.00 | 4 |
| White Ale | 11.2 | 18.90 | 173 | 05.00 | 3 |
| **Kona** | | | | | |
| Black Sand Porter | 12 | 16.70 | 199 | 06.80 | 4 |
| Castaway IPA | 12 | 19.60 | 214 | 07.00 | 4 |
| Duke's Blond Ale | 12 | 16.70 | 153 | 04.50 | 3 |
| Fire Rock Pale Ale | 12 | 13.59 | 186 | 06.00 | 4 |
| Golden Ale | 12 | 16.00 | 166 | 05.30 | 3 |
| Kula Hefeweizen | 12 | 15.50 | 170 | 05.60 | 3 |
| Lavaman Red Ale | 12 | 18.20 | 180 | 05.60 | 4 |

| | Oz | Carbs | Cal | Abv | Weight Watcher's POINTS® |
|---|---|---|---|---|---|
| Longboard Lager | 12 | 13.28 | 174 | 05.50 | 3 |
| Pacific Golden Ale | 12 | 11.51 | 158 | 05.50 | 3 |
| Pipeline Porter | 12 | 19.00 | 181 | 05.40 | 4 |
| Wailua Wheat | 12 | 13.20 | 158 | 05.40 | 3 |

## Kreuzberg Klosterbrauerei (Germany)

| | Oz | Carbs | Cal | Abv | Weight Watcher's POINTS® |
|---|---|---|---|---|---|
| Dunkel | 12 | 15.30 | 166 | 05.40 | 3 |
| Helles Hefe-Weizen | 12 | 14.10 | 165 | 05.60 | 3 |
| Pils | 12 | 14.10 | 165 | 05.60 | 3 |
| Weinachts-Bock | 12 | 22.10 | 236 | 07.60 | 5 |

## Kronenbourg (France)

| | Oz | Carbs | Cal | Abv | Weight Watcher's POINTS® |
|---|---|---|---|---|---|
| Kronenbourg 1664 | 12 | 16.33 | 156 | 05.00 | 3 |
| Kronenbourg 1664 Blanc | 12 | 14.91 | 168 | 05.00 | 3 |

## Labatt (Canada)

| | Oz | Carbs | Cal | Abv | Weight Watcher's POINTS® |
|---|---|---|---|---|---|
| Blue | 12 | 10.51 | 153 | 05.00 | 3 |
| Light | 12 | 07.90 | 111 | 04.00 | 2 |
| Sterling | ~11 | 02.50 | 088 | 04.00 | 2 |

## Lake Superior

| | Oz | Carbs | Cal | Abv | Weight Watcher's POINTS® |
|---|---|---|---|---|---|
| Mesabi Red | 12 | 21.10 | 211 | 06.50 | 4 |

## Latrobe (Canada)

| | Oz | Carbs | Cal | Abv | Weight Watcher's POINTS® |
|---|---|---|---|---|---|
| Rolling Green Light | 12 | 02.60 | 084 | 03.70 | 2 |
| Rolling Rock | 12 | 10.00 | 120 | 04.50 | 2 |

## Laurelwood

| | Oz | Carbs | Cal | Abv | Weight Watcher's POINTS® |
|---|---|---|---|---|---|
| Amber Ale | 12 | 17.20 | 168 | 05.10 | 3 |
| Boss IPA | 12 | 17.40 | 200 | 06.60 | 4 |
| Hooligan | 12 | 18.00 | 175 | 05.30 | 3 |
| Mother Lode Golden Ale | 12 | 14.90 | 157 | 05.10 | 3 |

| | Oz | Carbs | Cal | Abv | Weight Watcher's POINTS® |
|---|---|---|---|---|---|
| Organic Free Range Red | 12 | 18.50 | 188 | 05.90 | 4 |
| Organic Tree Hugger Porter | 12 | 18.50 | 186 | 05.80 | 4 |
| Piston Pale Ale | 12 | 15.60 | 174 | 05.60 | 3 |
| Space Stout | 12 | 23.25 | 215 | 06.10 | 4 |
| Workhorse IPA | 12 | 20.00 | 226 | 07.50 | 4 |

## Leffe (Belgium)

| | Oz | Carbs | Cal | Abv | |
|---|---|---|---|---|---|
| Blond | 12 | 17.75 | 217 | 06.60 | 4 |
| Brune | 12 | 18.82 | 217 | 06.50 | 4 |

## Left Hand

| | Oz | Carbs | Cal | Abv | |
|---|---|---|---|---|---|
| Black Jack Porter | 12 | 22.50 | 214 | 06.34 | 4 |
| Chainsaw Ale | 12 | 26.50 | 282 | 09.00 | 6 |
| Deep Cover Brown Ale | 12 | 17.50 | 155 | 04.23 | 3 |
| Haystack Wheat | 12 | 18.90 | 173 | 05.00 | 3 |
| Imperial Stout | 12 | 31.40 | 304 | 09.16 | 6 |
| Jackman's Pale Ale | 12 | 19.20 | 177 | 05.20 | 3 |
| JuJu Ginger | 12 | 12.10 | 131 | 04.38 | 3 |
| Milk Stout | 12 | 26.00 | 208 | 05.25 | 4 |
| Oktoberfest | 12 | 26.00 | 220 | 06.00 | 4 |
| Polestar Pilsner | 12 | 17.90 | 159 | 04.58 | 3 |
| Ryebock Lager | 12 | 27.80 | 258 | 07.60 | 5 |
| Sawtooth Ale | 12 | 18.80 | 162 | 04.48 | 3 |
| Snowbound Ale | 12 | 27.70 | 255 | 07.60 | 5 |
| Twin Sisters | 12 | 23.60 | 280 | 09.60 | 6 |

## Legend

| | Oz | Carbs | Cal | Abv | |
|---|---|---|---|---|---|
| Belgian Triple | 12 | 24.80 | 273 | 09.00 | 5 |
| Brown Ale | 12 | 19.20 | 197 | 06.30 | 4 |

|  | Oz | Carbs | Cal | Abv | Weight Watcher's POINTS® |
|---|---|---|---|---|---|
| Dopplebock | 12 | 24.60 | 253 | 07.90 | 5 |
| Golden IPA | 12 | 21.20 | 229 | 07.50 | 4 |
| Lager | 12 | 14.80 | 154 | 04.70 | 3 |
| Oktoberfest | 12 | 19.25 | 188 | 05.70 | 4 |
| Pilsner | 12 | 20.40 | 201 | 06.10 | 4 |
| Porter | 12 | 23.70 | 218 | 06.40 | 4 |
| Stout | 12 | 17.60 | 168 | 05.10 | 3 |

### Leinenkugel (See MillerCoors)

### Lily's Seafood Grill

| | Oz | Carbs | Cal | Abv | Weight Watcher's POINTS® |
|---|---|---|---|---|---|
| Light Pilsner | 12 | 11.70 | 137 | 04.70 | 3 |
| Reggie's French River Red | 12 | 17.30 | 181 | 05.80 | 4 |
| Strange Stout | 12 | 22.40 | 190 | 05.20 | 4 |
| Whitefish Bay Wheat | 12 | 14.60 | 159 | 05.20 | 3 |

### Lindemans (Belgium)

| | Oz | Carbs | Cal | Abv | Weight Watcher's POINTS® |
|---|---|---|---|---|---|
| Framboise Lambic | 12 | 34.40 | 183 | 02.30 | 4 |

### Lion-Nathan (AU,NZ)

| | Oz | Carbs | Cal | Abv | Weight Watcher's POINTS® |
|---|---|---|---|---|---|
| Amstel | 12 | 04.97 | 110 | 04.70 | 2 |
| Beck's (AU) | 12 | 09.23 | 151 | 05.00 | 3 |
| Black Mac | 12 | | 129 | 04.00 | 2 |
| Blond Mac | 12 | | 148 | 05.00 | 3 |
| Blue Bitter | 12 | 14.56 | 099 | 02.30 | 2 |
| Blue Ice | 12 | 08.88 | 092 | 02.30 | 2 |
| Boddington's | 12 | 12.78 | 144 | 04.80 | 3 |
| Canterbury Draught | 12 | 11.72 | 117 | 04.00 | 2 |
| Carbine Stout | 12 | 14.56 | 160 | 05.10 | 3 |
| Corona Extra (NZ) | 12 | | 148 | 04.60 | 3 |
| Emu Bitter | 12 | 12.43 | 142 | 04.50 | 3 |

|  | Oz | Carbs | Cal | Abv | Weight Watcher's POINTS® |
|---|---|---|---|---|---|
| Emu Draft | 12 | 09.94 | 107 | 03.00 | 2 |
| Emu Export | 12 | 09.59 | 131 | 04.50 | 3 |
| Emundi | 12 | 11.00 | 138 | 04.80 | 3 |
| Gold Bitter | 12 | 10.65 | 103 | 03.00 | 2 |
| Guinness Draught (NZ) | 12 | 05.33 | 133 | 04.20 | 3 |
| Gulf Lager | 12 | 09.23 | 103 | 03.20 | 2 |
| Hahn Premium | 12 | 11.20 | 241 | 05.00 | 5 |
| Hahn Premium Light | 12 | 11.00 | 099 | 02.70 | 2 |
| Hahn Super Dry | 12 | 03.20 | 179 | 04.60 | 3 |
| Heineken | 12 | 10.65 | 142 | 05.00 | 3 |
| Ice Beer | 12 | 08.17 | 110 | 04.00 | 2 |
| James Squire Original Amber Ale | 12 | 14.91 | 181 | 05.00 | 4 |
| James Squire Australian Strong | 12 | 17.34 | 209 | 06.80 | 4 |
| James Squire Golden Ale | 12 | 15.98 | 138 | 04.50 | 3 |
| James Squire IPA | 12 | 21.30 | 185 | 05.60 | 4 |
| James Squire Pilsener | 12 | 15.98 | 185 | 05.00 | 4 |
| James Squire Porter | 12 | 14.91 | 181 | 05.00 | 4 |
| Kilkenny | 12 |  | 128 | 04.30 | 2 |
| Kirin Ichiban | 12 | 11.36 | 099 | 05.00 | 2 |
| Knappstein Reserve Lager | 12 | 15.27 | 174 | 05.60 | 3 |
| Light Ice (AU) | 12 | 08.17 | 110 | 04.00 | 2 |
| Light Ice (NZ) | 12 | 06.75 | 082 | 02.50 | 2 |
| Lion Brown | 12 | 08.70 | 117 | 04.00 | 2 |

|  | Oz | Carbs | Cal | Abv | Weight Watcher's POINTS® |
|---|---|---|---|---|---|
| Lion Ice | 12 | 08.17 | 131 | 04.00 | 3 |
| Lion Pils | 12 |  | 121 | 04.00 | 2 |
| Lion Red | 12 | 09.23 | 117 | 04.00 | 2 |
| Mac's Copperhop | 12 |  | 149 | 05.00 | 3 |
| Mac's Gold (NZ) | 12 | 12.43 | 128 | 04.00 | 2 |
| Mac's Light | 12 |  | 041 | 01.00 | 1 |
| Mac's Nelson Reserve | 12 |  | 155 | 05.20 | 3 |
| Red Bitter | 12 | 12.14 | 128 | 04.00 | 2 |
| Rheineck | 12 | 12.00 | 089 | 03.50 | 2 |
| Southwark Bitter | 12 | 09.94 | 135 | 04.50 | 3 |
| Southwark Premium | 12 | 09.94 | 142 | 05.00 | 3 |
| Southwark Stout | 12 | 12.78 | 206 | 07.40 | 4 |
| Speight's Gold Medal | 12 | 08.88 | 114 | 04.00 | 2 |
| Speights Old Dark | 12 | 10.30 | 128 | 04.00 | 2 |
| Speight's Pale Ale | 12 | 11.30 | 135 | 04.50 | 3 |
| Steinlager | 12 | 08.52 | 138 | 05.00 | 3 |
| Steinlager (NZ) | 12 | 11.00 | 142 | 05.00 | 3 |
| Swan Draught | 12 | 09.59 | 131 | 04.50 | 3 |
| Swan Stout | 12 | 12.78 | 206 | 07.40 | 4 |
| Tooheys Gold Bitter | 12 | 10.83 | 103 | 03.00 | 2 |
| Tooheys Blue Ice | 12 | 08.88 | 092 | 02.50 | 2 |
| Tooheys Extra Dry | 12 | 08.88 | 135 | 05.00 | 3 |
| Tooheys Extra Dry Platinum | 12 | 11.72 | 178 | 06.50 | 3 |
| Tooheys Maxim | 12 | 05.68 | 107 | 04.60 | 2 |
| Tooheys New | 12 | 11.00 | 135 | 04.60 | 3 |
| Tooheys New White Stag | 12 | 03.20 | 179 | 04.60 | 3 |

|  | Oz | Carbs | Cal | Abv | Weight Watcher's POINTS® |
|---|---|---|---|---|---|
| Tooheys Old | 12 | 11.36 | 142 | 04.40 | 3 |
| Tooheys Pils | 12 | 06.75 | 121 | 04.50 | 2 |
| Waikato Draught | 12 | 07.10 | 110 | 04.00 | 2 |
| West End Draught | 12 | 08.52 | 128 | 04.50 | 2 |
| West End Export | 12 | 07.46 | 117 | 04.00 | 2 |
| West End Gold | 12 | 09.23 | 096 | 03.00 | 2 |
| West End Light | 12 | 07.46 | 089 | 02.30 | 2 |
| XXXX Bitter | 12 | 09.59 | 131 | 04.60 | 3 |
| XXXX DL Lager | 12 | 03.55 | 101 | 04.40 | 2 |
| XXX Light | 12 | 09.23 | 089 | 02.30 | 2 |
| XXXX Draught | 12 | 07.45 | 128 | 04.50 | 2 |
| XXXX Gold | 12 | 07.81 | 103 | 03.50 | 2 |
| XXX Special Brew | 12 | 14.56 | 181 | 06.50 | 4 |

## Long Beach

| | Oz | Carbs | Cal | Abv | |
|---|---|---|---|---|---|
| Thin Ice | 12 | 01.00 | 094 | 04.20 | 2 |

## Lost Coast

| | Oz | Carbs | Cal | Abv | |
|---|---|---|---|---|---|
| Winterbraun | 12 | 25.40 | 232 | 06.70 | 5 |

## Löwenbräu (Germany)

| | Oz | Carbs | Cal | Abv | |
|---|---|---|---|---|---|
| Alkoholfrei | 12 | 15.90 | 078 | <.50 | 1 |
| Dunkel | 12 | 14.50 | 165 | 05.50 | 3 |
| Original | 12 | 13.80 | 150 | 05.20 | 3 |
| Oktoberfestbier | 12 | 15.80 | 180 | 06.10 | 4 |
| Premium Pils | 12 | 13.80 | 150 | 05.20 | 3 |
| Triumphator | 12 | 25.10 | 245 | 07.60 | 5 |
| Urtyp | 12 | 15.00 | 160 | 05.40 | 3 |
| Weisse | 12 | 13.80 | 150 | 05.20 | 3 |

## Lucky Labrador

| | Oz | Carbs | Cal | Abv | |
|---|---|---|---|---|---|
| Best Bitter | 12 | 12.40 | 138 | 04.50 | 3 |

| | Oz | Carbs | Cal | Abv | Weight Watcher's POINTS® |
|---|---|---|---|---|---|
| Holiday Ale | 12 | 27.40 | 233 | 06.40 | 5 |
| IPA | 12 | 25.30 | 198 | 05.00 | 4 |
| OGA | 12 | 14.70 | 146 | 04.50 | 3 |
| Porter | 12 | 25.30 | 198 | 05.00 | 4 |
| Red | 12 | 19.30 | 175 | 05.00 | 3 |
| Rye | 12 | 18.40 | 161 | 04.50 | 3 |
| Stout | 12 | 26.60 | 232 | 06.50 | 5 |

## Mackeson (UK)

| | Oz | Carbs | Cal | Abv | Weight Watcher's POINTS® |
|---|---|---|---|---|---|
| Stout | 12 | 16.33 | 204 | 03.00 | 4 |

## Mad River

| | Oz | Carbs | Cal | Abv | Weight Watcher's POINTS® |
|---|---|---|---|---|---|
| Jamaica Red | 12 | 20.50 | 214 | 06.80 | 4 |
| Jamica Sunset IPA | 12 | 18.70 | 206 | 07.00 | 4 |
| John Barleycorn Barleywine | 12 | 30.00 | 321 | 09.80 | 6 |
| Steelhead Double IPA | 12 | 22.80 | 261 | 08.60 | 5 |
| Steelhead Extra Pale Ale | 12 | 16.70 | 180 | 05.90 | 4 |
| Steelhead Extra Stout | 12 | 25.90 | 233 | 06.60 | 5 |
| Steelhead Scotch Porter | 12 | 20.50 | 214 | 06.80 | 4 |
| Sunset IPA | 12 | 18.70 | 206 | 06.80 | 4 |

## Mayflower

| | Oz | Carbs | Cal | Abv | Weight Watcher's POINTS® |
|---|---|---|---|---|---|
| Golden Ale | 12 | 12.20 | 140 | 04.70 | 3 |
| IPA | 12 | 23.00 | 228 | 07.00 | 4 |
| Pale Ale | 12 | 17.00 | 163 | 04.90 | 3 |
| Porter | 12 | 21.80 | 194 | 05.50 | 4 |

## Max Lager's

| | Oz | Carbs | Cal | Abv | Weight Watcher's POINTS® |
|---|---|---|---|---|---|
| Black | 12 | 21.40 | 186 | 05.20 | 4 |

|  | Oz | Carbs | Cal | Abv | Weight Watcher's POINTS® |
|---|---|---|---|---|---|
| Bock | 12 | 24.20 | 260 | 08.50 | 5 |
| Gold | 12 | 15.80 | 170 | 05.50 | 3 |
| Oktoberfest | 12 | 23.90 | 222 | 06.50 | 4 |
| Red | 12 | 23.90 | 190 | 04.90 | 4 |

## McMenamins

|  | Oz | Carbs | Cal | Abv | Weight Watcher's POINTS® |
|---|---|---|---|---|---|
| Bagdad Ale | 12 | 12.00 | 146 | 05.03 | 3 |
| Black Rabbit Porter | 12 | 19.30 | 188 | 05.55 | 4 |
| Cascade Head | 12 | 09.80 | 129 | 04.52 | 2 |
| Crystal Ale | 12 | 15.20 | 164 | 05.16 | 3 |
| Edgefield Wheat | 12 | 12.50 | 147 | 04.77 | 3 |
| Hammerhead | 12 | 16.00 | 183 | 05.93 | 4 |
| Irish Stout | 12 | 12.00 | 143 | 04.77 | 3 |
| Kris Kringle | 12 | 18.70 | 191 | 05.81 | 4 |
| Nebraska Bitter | 12 | 12.50 | 143 | 04.64 | 3 |
| Ruby | 12 | 09.50 | 123 | 04.90 | 2 |
| Scarecrow ESB | 12 | 14.50 | 151 | 04.64 | 3 |
| Sleepy Hollow Nut Brown | 12 | 16.00 | 164 | 05.03 | 3 |
| Sunflower IPA | 12 | 17.70 | 203 | 06.71 | 4 |
| Terminator Stout | 12 | 22.00 | 215 | 06.45 | 4 |
| Workingman's Red | 12 | 14.50 | 154 | 04.77 | 3 |

## Metropolitan

|  | Oz | Carbs | Cal | Abv | Weight Watcher's POINTS® |
|---|---|---|---|---|---|
| Dynamo Copper | 12 | 18.20 | 181 | 05.60 | 4 |
| Flywheel | 12 | 20.10 | 176 | 05.00 | 3 |

## Middle Ages

|  | Oz | Carbs | Cal | Abv | Weight Watcher's POINTS® |
|---|---|---|---|---|---|
| Beast Bitter | 12 | 17.90 | 175 | 05.30 | 3 |
| Grail Ale | 12 | 17.50 | 165 | 04.90 | 3 |
| White Knight | 12 | 16.40 | 143 | 04.00 | 3 |

|  | Oz | Carbs | Cal | Abv | Weight Watcher's POINTS® |
|---|---|---|---|---|---|
| **MillerCoors** | | | | | |
| <u>Domestic Beers</u> | | | | | |
| Coors | 12 | 12.20 | 149 | 04.91 | 3 |
| Coors Light | 12 | 05.30 | 104 | 04.15 | 2 |
| Extra Gold Lager | 12 | 12.50 | 152 | 04.97 | 3 |
| Hamm's | 12 | 12.10 | 144 | 04.70 | 3 |
| Hamm's Golden Draft | 12 | 12.10 | 144 | 04.70 | 3 |
| Hamm's Special Light | 12 | 08.30 | 110 | 03.90 | 2 |
| Icehouse 5.0 | 12 | 08.70 | 132 | 05.00 | 3 |
| Icehouse 5.5 | 12 | 09.80 | 149 | 05.50 | 3 |
| Keystone Ice | 12 | 05.90 | 142 | 05.90 | 3 |
| Keystone Light | 12 | 05.50 | 123 | 04.13 | 2 |
| Keystone Premium | 12 | 05.80 | 111 | 04.43 | 2 |
| Magnum Malt Liquor | 12 | 11.20 | 157 | 05.60 | 3 |
| MGD 64 | 12 | 02.40 | 064 | 02.80 | 1 |
| Mickey's | 12 | 11.20 | 157 | 05.60 | 3 |
| Mickey's Ice | 12 | 11.80 | 157 | 05.80 | 3 |
| Miller Chill | 12 | 06.50 | 110 | 04.20 | 2 |
| Miller Genuine Draft | 12 | 13.10 | 143 | 04.70 | 3 |
| Miller High Life | 12 | 13.10 | 143 | 04.70 | 3 |
| Miller HL Light | 12 | 07.00 | 110 | 04.20 | 2 |
| Miller Lite | 12 | 03.20 | 096 | 04.20 | 2 |
| Milwaukee's Best | 12 | 11.40 | 128 | 04.30 | 2 |
| Milwaukee's Best Ice | 12 | 07.30 | 144 | 05.90 | 3 |
| Milwaukee's Best Light | 12 | 03.50 | 098 | 04.20 | 2 |

|  | Oz | Carbs | Cal | Abv | Weight Watcher's POINTS® |
|---|---|---|---|---|---|
| Olde English 800 | 12 | 10.50 | 160 | 05.90 | 3 |
| Olde English 800 7.5 | 12 | 13.40 | 202 | 07.50 | 4 |
| Olde English High Gravity 800 | 12 | 14.70 | 220 | 08.00 | 4 |
| Red Dog | 12 | 14.10 | 147 | 08.00 | 3 |
| Southpaw Light | 12 | 06.60 | 123 | 05.00 | 2 |
| Steel Reserve High Gravity | 12 | 16.00 | 222 | 08.10 | 4 |
| Steel Reserve Triple Export 8.1% | 12 | 16.00 | 222 | 08.10 | 4 |
| Steel Six | 12 | 11.00 | 160 | 06.00 | 3 |
| Imports |  |  |  |  |  |
| Águila | 12 | 10.40 | 122 | 03.90 | 2 |
| Cristal | 12 | 11.60 | 134 | 04.50 | 3 |
| Cusqueña | 12 | 12.00 | 140 | 04.80 | 3 |
| Grolsch Amber Ale | 12 | 12.20 | 160 | 05.40 | 3 |
| Grolsch Blond Lager | 12 | 12.20 | 120 | 02.80 | 2 |
| Grolsch Light Lager | 12 | 05.70 | 097 | 03.60 | 2 |
| Grolsch Premium Lager | 12 | 10.40 | 147 | 05.00 | 3 |
| Lech | 12 | 10.40 | 143 | 04.90 | 3 |
| Molson Canadian | 12 | 11.10 | 136 | 05.00 | 3 |
| Molson Canadian Light | 12 | 09.90 | 113 | 03.90 | 2 |
| Molson Golden | 12 | 10.90 | 133 | 05.00 | 3 |
| Molson Ice | 12 | 11.60 | 160 | 05.60 | 3 |
| Molson XXX | 12 | 10.90 | 201 | 07.30 | 4 |
| Peroni Nastro Azzurro | 12 | 11.40 | 150 | 05.10 | 3 |
| Pilsner Urquell | 12 | 16.00 | 156 | 04.40 | 3 |

| | Oz | Carbs | Cal | Abv | Weight Watcher's POINTS® |
|---|---|---|---|---|---|
| Tyskie | 12 | 10.60 | 153 | 05.40 | 3 |

Craft

| | Oz | Carbs | Cal | Abv | Weight Watcher's POINTS® |
|---|---|---|---|---|---|
| Blue Moon Belgian Ale | 12 | 13.00 | 164 | 05.36 | 3 |
| Blue Moon Full Moon | 12 | 15.30 | 180 | 05.52 | 4 |
| Blue Moon Harvest Moon Pumpkin Ale | 12 | 14.70 | 180 | 05.76 | 4 |
| Blue Moon Honey Moon Summer Ale | 12 | 12.50 | 157 | 05.12 | 3 |
| Blue Moon Rising Moon Spring Ale | 12 | 11.90 | 161 | 05.40 | 3 |
| Frederick Miller Classic Chocolate Lager | 12 | 18.40 | 195 | 05.50 | 4 |
| Henry Weinhard's Belgian Style Wheat | 12 | 13.30 | 155 | 04.90 | 3 |
| Henry Weinhard's Blonde | 12 | 14.00 | 161 | 05.10 | 3 |
| Henry Weinhard's Blue Boar | 12 | 13.00 | 147 | 04.60 | 3 |
| Henry Weinhard's Classic Dark Lager | 12 | 16.00 | 164 | 05.00 | 3 |
| Henry Weinhard's Hefeweizen | 12 | 12.10 | 151 | 04.90 | 3 |
| Henry Weinhard's India Pale Ale | 12 | 16.40 | 189 | 06.00 | 4 |
| Henry Weinhard's Private Reserve | 12 | 09.90 | 150 | 04.80 | 3 |
| Henry Weinhard's Summer Wheat Ale | 12 | 13.30 | 155 | 04.90 | 3 |
| Leinenkugel's Apple Spice | 12 | 26.80 | 208 | 04.90 | 4 |

|  | Oz | Carbs | Cal | Abv | Weight Watcher's POINTS® |
|---|---|---|---|---|---|
| Leinenkugel's Berry Weiss | 12 | 28.00 | 207 | 04.70 | 4 |
| Leinenkugel's BIG BUTT Dopplebock | 12 | 18.80 | 195 | 05.80 | 4 |
| Leinenkugel's Creamy Dark | 12 | 16.80 | 170 | 04.90 | 3 |
| Leinenkugel's Fireside Nut Brown | 12 | 13.40 | 130 | 04.90 | 3 |
| Leinenkugel's Honey Weiss | 12 | 12.00 | 149 | 04.90 | 3 |
| Leinenkugel's Light | 12 | 05.80 | 109 | 04.20 | 2 |
| Leinenkugel's Oktoberfest Lager | 12 | 17.80 | 170 | 05.10 | 3 |
| Leinenkugel's Original Lager | 12 | 13.90 | 152 | 04.70 | 3 |
| Leinenkugel's Red Lager | 12 | 16.20 | 166 | 04.90 | 3 |
| Leinenkugel's Summer Shandy | 12 | 12.00 | 130 | 04.20 | 3 |
| Leinenkugel's Sunset Wheat | 12 | 16.00 | 165 | 04.90 | 3 |
| Sheaf Stout | 12 | 18.80 | 188 | 05.80 | 4 |

## Specialties

|  | Oz | Carbs | Cal | Abv | Weight Watcher's POINTS® |
|---|---|---|---|---|---|
| Coors NA | 12 | 14.80 | 066 | 00.50 | 1 |
| Foster's | 12 | 11.20 | 145 | 05.00 | 3 |
| Foster's Premium Ale | 12 | 12.50 | 160 | 05.50 | 3 |
| George Killian's Irish Red | 12 | 14.80 | 162 | 04.98 | 3 |
| Sharp's | 12 | 12.10 | 058 | 00.40 | 1 |
| Sparks | 12 | 35.00 | 257 | 06.00 | 5 |

| | Oz | Carbs | Cal | Abv | Weight Watcher's POINTS® |
|---|---|---|---|---|---|
| Sparks Light | 12 | 03.80 | 133 | 06.00 | 3 |
| Sparks Plus 6% | 12 | 35.00 | 258 | 06.00 | 5 |
| Sparks Plus 7% | 12 | 37.00 | 288 | 07.00 | 6 |
| Winterfest | 12 | 17.40 | 185 | 05.64 | 4 |
| Zima | 12 | 22.10 | 184 | 04.94 | 4 |
| Zima Pineapple Citrus | 12 | 21.70 | 182 | 04.94 | 4 |
| Zima Tangerine | 12 | 21.60 | 181 | 04.94 | 4 |

## Millstream

| | Oz | Carbs | Cal | Abv | Weight Watcher's POINTS® |
|---|---|---|---|---|---|
| German Pilsner | 12 | 14.90 | 148 | 04.90 | 3 |
| Schild Brau Amber | 12 | 16.80 | 167 | 05.70 | 3 |
| Millstream Wheat | 12 | 11.00 | 137 | 04.50 | 3 |

## Minhas Craft

| | Oz | Carbs | Cal | Abv | Weight Watcher's POINTS® |
|---|---|---|---|---|---|
| 1845 Pils | 12 | 09.90 | 160 | 05.50 | 3 |
| Clear Creek Ice | 12 | 15.70 | 182 | 06.20 | 4 |
| Fighting Bill Bock | 12 | 11.70 | 160 | 05.50 | 3 |
| Huber | 12 | 14.20 | 142 | 04.45 | 3 |
| Huber Bock | 12 | 20.80 | 189 | 05.40 | 4 |
| KickAxe | 12 | 10.00 | 211 | 08.60 | 4 |
| Lazy Mutt | 12 | 14.10 | 154 | 05.00 | 3 |
| Minhas Light | 12 | 08.50 | 097 | 03.60 | 2 |
| Mountain Creek | 12 | 16.30 | 165 | 05.50 | 3 |
| Rhinelander | 12 | 14.30 | 141 | 04.50 | 3 |
| Swiss Amber | 12 | 09.90 | 158 | 05.50 | 3 |
| WI Club | 12 | 12.70 | 139 | 04.80 | 3 |

## Montheith's (New Zealand)

| | Oz | Carbs | Cal | Abv | Weight Watcher's POINTS® |
|---|---|---|---|---|---|
| Black Beer | 12 | 16.90 | 168 | 05.20 | 3 |
| Celtic Beer | 12 | 13.20 | 138 | 04.40 | 3 |

|  | Oz | Carbs | Cal | Abv | Weight Watcher's POINTS® |
|---|---|---|---|---|---|
| Dopplebock | 12 | 21.90 | 216 | 06.60 | 4 |
| Golden Lager | 12 | 11.60 | 143 | 05.00 | 3 |
| Original Ale | 12 | 12.70 | 128 | 04.00 | 2 |
| Pilsner | 12 | 14.30 | 154 | 05.00 | 3 |
| Radler | 12 | 16.20 | 162 | 05.00 | 3 |
| Summer Ale | 12 | 15.30 | 158 | 05.00 | 3 |

### Moosehead (Canada)

|  | Oz | Carbs | Cal | Abv | |
|---|---|---|---|---|---|
| Alpine Lager | 11 | 10.80 | 141 | 05.00 | 3 |
| Alpine Light | 11 | 08.73 | 115 | 04.00 | 2 |
| Dry | 11 | 11.60 | 153 | 05.50 | 3 |

### Mountain Sun

|  | Oz | Carbs | Cal | Abv | |
|---|---|---|---|---|---|
| Annapurna Amber | 12 | 20.30 | 198 | 06.00 | 4 |
| Brown Ale | 12 | 17.50 | 165 | 04.90 | 3 |
| Chazz Cat Rye | 12 | 15.10 | 183 | 06.30 | 4 |
| Chocolate Stout | 12 | 27.00 | 230 | 06.30 | 5 |
| Dopplebock | 12 | 28.30 | 271 | 08.10 | 5 |
| Golden Ale | 12 | 15.70 | 164 | 05.25 | 3 |
| Kind Ale | 12 | 17.20 | 190 | 06.30 | 4 |
| Kolsch | 12 | 14.20 | 163 | 05.50 | 3 |
| Java Porter | 12 | 18.50 | 191 | 06.00 | 4 |
| Raspberry Wheat | 12 | 12.40 | 156 | 05.50 | 3 |
| Scotch Ale | 12 | 26.10 | 257 | 07.90 | 5 |
| XXX Pale Ale | 12 | 22.10 | 236 | 07.60 | 5 |

### Mönchshof (Germany)

|  | Oz | Carbs | Cal | Abv | |
|---|---|---|---|---|---|
| Bockbier | 12 | 22.40 | 223 | 06.90 | 4 |
| Kellerbier | 12 | 14.80 | 164 | 05.40 | 3 |
| Lager | 12 | 14.40 | 152 | 04.90 | 3 |
| Landbier | 12 | 14.80 | 164 | 05.40 | 3 |

| | Oz | Carbs | Cal | Abv | Weight Watcher's POINTS® |
|---|---|---|---|---|---|
| Original | 12 | 14.50 | 153 | 04.90 | 3 |
| Schwarzbier | 12 | 17.50 | 166 | 04.90 | 3 |
| Weinachtsbier | 12 | 17.40 | 179 | 05.60 | 3 |
| **Murphy (Ireland)** | | | | | |
| Murphy's Irish Red Beer | 12 | 11.00 | 171 | 05.00 | 3 |
| Murphy's Stout | 12 | 09.00 | 149 | 04.00 | 3 |
| **Natty Greene's** | | | | | |
| Amber Ale | 12 | 20.00 | 172 | 04.80 | 3 |
| Brown Ale | 12 | 21.00 | 169 | 04.40 | 3 |
| Golden Ale | 12 | 12.00 | 122 | 03.80 | 2 |
| Pale Ale | 12 | 17.90 | 173 | 05.30 | 3 |
| Stout | 12 | 12.40 | 138 | 04.50 | 3 |
| **New Belgium** | | | | | |
| 1554 | 12 | 25.00 | 160 | 05.20 | 3 |
| 2 Below | 12 | 17.00 | 200 | 06.60 | 4 |
| Abbey | 12 | 18.00 | 200 | 07.00 | 4 |
| Abbey Grand Cru | 12 | 21.00 | 270 | 09.50 | 5 |
| Bens Saison | 12 | 21.00 | 190 | 05.30 | 4 |
| Bier de Mars | 12 | 20.10 | 195 | 06.20 | 4 |
| Blue Paddle | 12 | 14.00 | 140 | 04.80 | 3 |
| Eric's Ale | 12 | 19.00 | 220 | 07.00 | 4 |
| Fat Tire | 12 | 15.00 | 160 | 05.20 | 3 |
| Frambozen | 12 | 19.60 | 200 | 06.50 | 4 |
| Giddy Up | 12 | 15.00 | 180 | 06.00 | 4 |
| La Folie | 12 | 09.00 | 200 | 06.00 | 4 |
| La Terroir | 12 | 09.00 | 200 | 06.00 | 4 |
| Mighty Arrow | 12 | 15.50 | 180 | 06.00 | 4 |

| | Oz | Carbs | Cal | Abv | Weight Watcher's POINTS® |
|---|---|---|---|---|---|
| Mothership Wit | 12 | 15.00 | 155 | 04.80 | 3 |
| Old Cherry | 12 | 17.50 | 200 | 06.50 | 4 |
| Skinny Dip | 12 | 07.00 | 110 | 04.20 | 2 |
| Sunshine Wheat | 12 | 12.80 | 145 | 04.80 | 2 |
| Trippel | 12 | 20.00 | 215 | 07.80 | 4 |

### New Century

| | Oz | Carbs | Cal | Abv | Weight Watcher's POINTS® |
|---|---|---|---|---|---|
| Edison Light | 12 | 06.60 | 109 | 04.00 | 2 |

### New Glarus

| | Oz | Carbs | Cal | Abv | Weight Watcher's POINTS® |
|---|---|---|---|---|---|
| Spotted Cow | 12 | 13.56 | 150 | 05.10 | 3 |

### New Holland

| | Oz | Carbs | Cal | Abv | Weight Watcher's POINTS® |
|---|---|---|---|---|---|
| Full Circle Single Malt | 12 | 14.75 | 160 | 05.20 | 3 |
| Ichabod Pumpkin Ale | 12 | 17.25 | 186 | 06.10 | 4 |
| Mad Hatter IPA | 12 | 16.70 | 165 | 05.10 | 3 |
| Paleooza Pale Ale | 12 | 17.75 | 187 | 06.00 | 4 |
| Poet Oatmeal Stout | 12 | 22.00 | 217 | 06.70 | 4 |
| Sundog Amber | 12 | 17.75 | 187 | 06.00 | 4 |
| Zoomer Wit | 12 | 15.00 | 161 | 05.20 | 3 |

### Nor'Wester (Saxer)

| | Oz | Carbs | Cal | Abv | Weight Watcher's POINTS® |
|---|---|---|---|---|---|
| Dunkel Weizen | 12 | 16.10 | 166 | 05.30 | 3 |
| Hefeweizen | 12 | 12.60 | 158 | 05.30 | 3 |
| Mt. Angel Oktoberfest | 12 | 23.70 | 217 | 06.30 | 4 |
| OPA | 12 | 19.30 | 186 | 05.70 | 4 |
| Raspberry Weizen | 12 | 12.60 | 158 | 05.30 | 3 |
| Smith Rock Bock | 12 | 23.70 | 217 | 06.30 | 4 |

### O'Keefe (Canada)

| | Oz | Carbs | Cal | Abv | Weight Watcher's POINTS® |
|---|---|---|---|---|---|
| Canadian Beer | 12 | | 142 | 04.90 | 3 |

| | Oz | Carbs | Cal | Abv | Weight Watcher's POINTS® |
|---|---|---|---|---|---|
| **Old Dominion** | | | | | |
| Domion Lager | 12 | 19.70 | 188 | 05.60 | 4 |
| **Orlando Brewing (Organic)** | | | | | |
| Blonde Ale | 12 | 10.60 | 130 | 04.50 | 3 |
| Pale Ale | 12 | 18.40 | 185 | 05.70 | 4 |
| **Pabst** | | | | | |
| Ballantine Ale | 12 | 15.90 | 174 | 05.70 | 3 |
| Blatz | 12 | 12.50 | 153 | 04.50 | 3 |
| Blatz Light | 12 | 08.30 | 094 | 03.50 | 2 |
| Carling Black Label | 12 | 12.50 | 138 | 04.40 | 3 |
| Champale Extra Dry | 12 | 06.20 | | | |
| Champale Golden | 12 | 12.70 | | | |
| Colt 45 | 12 | 11.10 | 174 | 06.10 | 3 |
| Falstaff | 12 | 11.90 | 163 | 05.10 | 3 |
| Heidelburg | 12 | 12.50 | 146 | 04.60 | 3 |
| Kingsbury NA | 12 | 11.50 | 056 | 00.40 | 1 |
| Lone Star | 12 | 11.40 | 145 | 04.70 | 3 |
| Lone Star Light | 12 | 08.30 | 113 | 03.90 | 2 |
| Lucky Lager | 12 | 11.90 | 146 | 04.70 | 3 |
| McSorley's Ale | 12 | 15.00 | 182 | 05.90 | 4 |
| McSorley's Black and Tan | 12 | 14.50 | 179 | 05.60 | 3 |
| National Bohemian | 12 | 11.40 | 135 | 04.30 | 3 |
| Old Milwaukee | 12 | 12.90 | 146 | 04.90 | 3 |
| Old Milwaukee Light | 12 | 08.30 | 119 | 03.80 | 2 |
| Old Style | 12 | 12.00 | 143 | 04.70 | 3 |
| Old Style Light | 12 | 07.00 | 113 | 04.20 | 2 |
| Olympia | 12 | 11.90 | 146 | 04.70 | 3 |

| | Oz | Carbs | Cal | Abv | Weight Watcher's POINTS® |
|---|---|---|---|---|---|
| Pabst | 12 | 12.10 | 153 | 05.00 | 3 |
| Pabst Light | 12 | 08.30 | 072 | 03.90 | 1 |
| Pabst NA | 12 | 12.00 | 057 | <0.50 | 1 |
| Pearl | 12 | 11.90 | 146 | 04.70 | 3 |
| Piels | 12 | 08.70 | 142 | 04.50 | 3 |
| Rainier | 12 | 11.40 | 143 | 04.70 | 3 |
| Schaefer | 12 | 12.00 | 142 | 04.60 | 3 |
| Schaefer's Light | 12 | 08.30 | 111 | 03.60 | 2 |
| Schlitz | 12 | 12.10 | 146 | 04.70 | 3 |
| Schmidt | 12 | 12.50 | 146 | 04.60 | 3 |
| Special Export | 12 | 12.10 | 145 | 04.60 | 3 |
| Stag | 12 | 12.50 | 145 | 04.60 | 3 |
| St. Ides | 12 | 10.60 | 163 | 05.90 | 3 |
| Stroh | 12 | 12.00 | 153 | 04.60 | 3 |
| Stroh Light | 12 | 07.00 | 114 | 03.82 | 2 |

## Papago

| | Oz | Carbs | Cal | Abv | Weight Watcher's POINTS® |
|---|---|---|---|---|---|
| El Robusto Porter | 12 | 19.60 | 241 | 08.40 | 5 |
| Elsies Coffee Milk Stout | 12 | 22.80 | 169 | 04.00 | 3 |
| Hop Dog | 12 | 21.00 | 223 | 07.20 | 4 |
| Hopfather Double IPA | 12 | 21.30 | 245 | 08.30 | 5 |
| Orange Blossom | 12 | 20.40 | 157 | 03.90 | 3 |
| Ryans Red | 12 | 20.20 | 176 | 04.90 | 3 |

## Paulaner (Germany)

| | Oz | Carbs | Cal | Abv | Weight Watcher's POINTS® |
|---|---|---|---|---|---|
| Hefe-Weissbier Alcoholfrei | 12 | | 050 | 00.00 | 1 |
| Hefe-Weissbier | 12 | 14.50 | 160 | 05.50 | 3 |

| | Oz | Carbs | Cal | Abv | Weight Watcher's POINTS® |
|---|---|---|---|---|---|
| Hefe-Weissbier Kristallklar | 12 | 11.80 | 150 | 05.50 | 3 |
| Hefe-Weissbier Dunkel | 12 | 15.20 | 160 | 05.30 | XX |
| Hefe-Weissbier Leicht | 12 | 09.50 | 104 | 03.20 | 2 |
| Müncher Diät Bier | 12 | 06.20 | 100 | 04.30 | 2 |
| Müncher Dunkel | 12 | 17.30 | 165 | 05.00 | 3 |
| Müncher Hell | 12 | 14.20 | 148 | 04.90 | 3 |
| Müncher Hell Leicht | 12 | 09.50 | 104 | 03.20 | 2 |
| Müncher Urtyp | 12 | 14.50 | 160 | 05.50 | 3 |
| Premium Pils | 12 | 14.20 | 145 | 04.90 | 3 |
| Oktoberfest | 12 | 16.40 | 180 | 06.00 | 4 |
| Salvator | 12 | 23.60 | 245 | 07.90 | 5 |

## Pete's Wicked

| | Oz | Carbs | Cal | Abv | Weight Watcher's POINTS® |
|---|---|---|---|---|---|
| Helles Lager | 12 | 14.60 | 163 | 05.00 | 3 |
| Honey Wheat | 12 | 16.30 | | | |
| Oktoberfest | 12 | 16.50 | 189 | 05.80 | 4 |
| Red Rush | 12 | 14.80 | 170 | 05.30 | 3 |
| Signature Pilsner | 12 | 13.90 | | | |
| Strawberry Blonde | 12 | 13.70 | 160 | 05.00 | 3 |
| Summer Brew | 12 | 14.20 | 163 | 04.70 | 3 |
| Wicked Ale | 12 | 15.30 | 174 | 05.30 | 3 |
| Winter Brew | 12 | 17.70 | 170 | 05.30 | 3 |

## Picaroons (Canada)

| | Oz | Carbs | Cal | Abv | Weight Watcher's POINTS® |
|---|---|---|---|---|---|
| Best Bitter | 12 | 19.00 | 166 | 04.70 | 3 |
| Blonde Ale | 12 | 20.00 | 164 | 04.30 | 3 |
| Dark & Stormy | 12 | 21.00 | 177 | 04.80 | 3 |
| Irish Red | 12 | 23.10 | 160 | 03.50 | 3 |

|  | Oz | Carbs | Cal | Abv | Weight Watcher's POINTS® |
|---|---|---|---|---|---|
| Man's Best Friend | 12 | 24.20 | 182 | 04.40 | 4 |
| Winter Warmer | 12 | 29.50 | 247 | 06.70 | 5 |
| Yippee IPA | 12 | 23.60 | 216 | 06.30 | 4 |
| **Pike** | | | | | |
| Barley Wine | 12 | 30.40 | 315 | 10.00 | 6 |
| Bride Ale | 12 | 18.90 | 173 | 05.00 | 3 |
| Double Ale | 12 | 24.00 | 231 | 07.00 | 5 |
| Extra Stout | 12 | 26.70 | 242 | 07.00 | 5 |
| Holiday Ale | 12 | 18.90 | 173 | 05.00 | 3 |
| Naughty Nellie | 12 | 17.20 | 159 | 04.70 | 3 |
| Pike Pale | 12 | 19.90 | 173 | 05.00 | 3 |
| Ruby Ale | 12 | 21.10 | 211 | 06.50 | 4 |
| Special Bitter | 12 | 19.80 | 192 | 05.80 | 4 |
| Tripel Ale | 12 | 17.00 | 242 | 09.00 | 5 |
| Wheat Ale | 12 | 16.10 | 152 | 04.50 | 3 |
| **Pilsner Urquell (Czech)** | | | | | |
| Pilsner Urquell | 12 | 15.70 | 160 | 04.30 | 3 |
| **Pittsburgh** | | | | | |
| Augustiner | 12 | 10.00 | 135 | 04.30 | 3 |
| Iron City | 12 | 10.00 | 140 | 04.50 | 3 |
| Iron City Light | 12 | 02.80 | 095 | 04.20 | 2 |
| **Pony Express** | | | | | |
| Gold Beer | 12 | 16.85 | 160 | 04.70 | 3 |
| Original Wheat | 12 | 17.90 | 174 | 04.90 | 3 |
| Rattlesnake Pale Ale | 12 | 13.85 | 174 | 04.90 | 3 |
| **Portland** | | | | | |
| Benchmark Old Ale | 12 | 32.10 | 316 | 09.40 | 6 |

| | Oz | Carbs | Cal | Abv | Weight Watcher's POINTS® |
|---|---|---|---|---|---|
| Black Watch Cream Porter | 12 | 20.80 | 189 | 05.30 | 4 |
| Bobby Dazzler Holiday Ale | 12 | 25.25 | 229 | 06.80 | 4 |
| Highlander Pale | 12 | 17.30 | 159 | 04.70 | 3 |
| Mac Frost | 12 | 23.25 | 225 | 06.70 | 4 |
| MacTarnahan's Amber Ale | 12 | 18.50 | 167 | 05.00 | 3 |
| Oregon Honey | 12 | 13.65 | 143 | 04.70 | 3 |
| Otto's Weiss | 12 | 17.45 | 167 | 04.90 | 3 |
| Portland Ale | 12 | 18.10 | 159 | 04.70 | 3 |
| Uncle Otto's Oktoberfest | 12 | 23.70 | 217 | 06.30 | 4 |
| Woodstock IPA | 12 | 20.35 | 207 | 06.50 | 4 |
| Zig Zag River Lager | 12 | 18.20 | 166 | 04.90 | 3 |

**Port Townsend**

| | Oz | Carbs | Cal | Abv | Weight Watcher's POINTS® |
|---|---|---|---|---|---|
| Barley Wine | 12 | 27.40 | 313 | 10.50 | 6 |
| Boatyard Bitter | 12 | 15.20 | 164 | 05.30 | 3 |
| Brown Porter | 12 | 19.20 | 185 | 05.60 | 4 |
| Chet's Gold | 12 | 11.80 | 156 | 05.60 | 3 |
| IPA | 12 | 16.80 | 190 | 06.30 | 4 |
| Pale Ale | 12 | 16.10 | 152 | 04.50 | 3 |
| Reel Amber | 12 | 16.00 | 164 | 05.20 | 3 |
| Scotch Ale | 12 | 21.40 | 220 | 07.00 | 4 |
| Strait Stout | 12 | 21.70 | 199 | 05.80 | 4 |
| Winter Ale | 12 | 23.60 | 237 | 07.40 | 5 |

**Pyramid**

| | Oz | Carbs | Cal | Abv | Weight Watcher's POINTS® |
|---|---|---|---|---|---|
| Apricot Weizen | 12 | 12.40 | 170 | 05.10 | 3 |
| Broken Rake | 12 | 24.50 | 200 | 06.10 | 4 |

|  | Oz | Carbs | Cal | Abv | Weight Watcher's POINTS® |
|---|---|---|---|---|---|
| Crystal | 12 | 15.10 | 160 | 05.30 | 3 |
| Hefeweizen | 12 | 16.40 | 166 | 05.20 | 3 |
| Snowcap Ale | 12 | 24.50 | 225 | 07.00 | 4 |
| Thunderhead | 12 | 24.10 | 225 | 06.70 | 4 |

## Real Ale Brewing Company

|  | Oz | Carbs | Cal | Abv | Weight Watcher's POINTS® |
|---|---|---|---|---|---|
| Brewhouse Brown Ale | 12 | 17.70 | 175 | 05.40 | 3 |
| Devil's Backbone | 12 | 21.90 | 244 | 08.10 | 5 |
| Dunkelroggen | 12 | 14.60 | 159 | 05.20 | 3 |
| Firemans #4 Blonde Ale | 12 | 15.00 | 160 | 05.10 | 3 |
| Full Moon Pale Rye Ale | 12 | 19.30 | 188 | 05.70 | 4 |
| Lost Gold IPA | 12 | 18.50 | 202 | 06.60 | 4 |
| Rio Blanco Pale Ale | 12 | 16.10 | 167 | 05.30 | 3 |
| Roggenbier | 12 | 19.20 | 171 | 04.90 | 3 |
| Shade Grown Coffee Porter | 12 | 19.80 | 189 | 05.60 | 4 |
| Sisyphus Barleywine Ale | 12 | 32.20 | 338 | 10.80 | 7 |

## ReaperAle (GreenFlash)

|  | Oz | Carbs | Cal | Abv | Weight Watcher's POINTS® |
|---|---|---|---|---|---|
| Deathly Pale Ale | 12 | 16.25 | 186 | 06.30 | 4 |
| Mortality Stout | 12 | 23.40 | 243 | 07.70 | 5 |
| Redemption Red Ale | 12 | 20.35 | 210 | 06.70 | 4 |

## Redhook

|  | Oz | Carbs | Cal | Abv | Weight Watcher's POINTS® |
|---|---|---|---|---|---|
| Blonde | 12 | 12.08 | 162 | 05.41 | 3 |
| Copperhook | 12 | 13.00 | 174 | 05.70 | 3 |
| ESB | 12 | 13.30 | 179 | 05.80 | 3 |
| Sun Rye | 12 | 07.12 | 131 | 04.70 | 3 |
| Blackhook Porter | 12 | 12.92 | 163 | 05.23 | 3 |

|  | Oz | Carbs | Cal | Abv | Weight Watcher's POINTS® |
|---|---|---|---|---|---|
| IPA | 12 | 12.23 | 186 | 06.51 | 4 |
| Late Harvest | 12 | 18.40 | 190 | 05.70 | 4 |
| Nut Brown Ale | 12 | 16.02 | 181 | 05.57 | 4 |
| Winter Hook | 12 | 14.92 | 175 | 05.52 | 3 |
| **Richbrau** | | | | | |
| Big Nasty Porter | 12 | 15.30 | 198 | 07.10 | 4 |
| Griffin Golden Ale | 12 | 10.40 | 148 | 05.60 | 3 |
| Old Nick Pale Ale | 12 | 12.20 | 158 | 05.60 | 3 |
| **Robert Simpson** | | | | | |
| Confederation Ale | 12 | 12.10 | 151 | 05.00 | 3 |
| **Rockfish Grill** | | | | | |
| Amber | 12 | 24.40 | 195 | 05.00 | 4 |
| Belgian Wit | 12 | 17.90 | 159 | 04.50 | 3 |
| Cream Ale | 12 | 24.00 | 216 | 06.20 | 4 |
| Doppelbock | 12 | 30.50 | 285 | 08.40 | 6 |
| ESB | 12 | 27.10 | 227 | 06.10 | 4 |
| Hefeweizen | 12 | 19.40 | 167 | 04.60 | 3 |
| Helles Fest Lager | 12 | 18.20 | 166 | 04.80 | 3 |
| Imperial Stout | 12 | 32.50 | 295 | 08.50 | 6 |
| IPA | 12 | 27.10 | 227 | 06.10 | 4 |
| Klosterbier | 12 | 20.70 | 186 | 05.30 | 4 |
| Maibock | 12 | 26.60 | 233 | 06.50 | 5 |
| Marzen | 12 | 27.40 | 233 | 06.40 | 5 |
| Oktoberfest | 12 | 29.20 | 241 | 06.40 | 5 |
| Pilsner | 12 | 20.80 | 180 | 05.00 | 4 |
| Porter | 12 | 21.20 | 174 | 04.60 | 3 |
| Red Ale | 12 | 23.50 | 175 | 04.20 | 3 |
| Scottish Ale | 12 | 35.00 | 300 | 08.30 | 6 |

| | Oz | Carbs | Cal | Abv | Weight Watcher's POINTS® |
|---|---|---|---|---|---|
| Stout | 12 | 26.30 | 202 | 05.00 | 4 |
| Vienna | 12 | 21.90 | 181 | 04.80 | 4 |
| Winter Ale | 12 | 28.50 | 250 | 07.00 | 5 |
| **Rocky River** | | | | | |
| American Alt | 12 | 25.30 | 189 | 04.50 | 4 |
| Blitzen Berry | 12 | 28.30 | 191 | 04.00 | 4 |
| Chocosaurus | 12 | 31.20 | 236 | 05.70 | 5 |
| Christmas Ale | 12 | 29.70 | 235 | 06.00 | 5 |
| Cupid's Revenge | 12 | 23.60 | 200 | 05.50 | 4 |
| Gold Kolsch | 12 | 21.00 | 161 | 04.00 | 3 |
| Hop Goblin | 12 | 29.40 | 259 | 07.30 | 5 |
| Irish Stout | 12 | 25.80 | 177 | 03.80 | 3 |
| Lakeshore Electric | 12 | 26.00 | 189 | 04.40 | 4 |
| Lil Warrior | 12 | 26.00 | 189 | 04.40 | 4 |
| Liquid Sunshine | 12 | 25.70 | 183 | 04.10 | 4 |
| Northern Lights | 12 | 27.10 | 196 | 04.50 | 4 |
| Pirate Light | 12 | 15.50 | 133 | 03.70 | 3 |
| Pumpkin Ale | 12 | 26.00 | 189 | 04.40 | 4 |
| Solstice Weiss | 12 | 27.60 | 190 | 04.10 | 4 |
| Subchaser Hefe | 12 | 26.40 | 190 | 04.30 | 4 |
| St Festivus | 12 | 26.60 | 202 | 04.90 | 4 |
| Summer Ale | 12 | 19.70 | 151 | 03.70 | 3 |
| **Rogue** | | | | | |
| American Amber | 12 | 16.00 | 173 | 05.60 | 3 |
| Brutal Bitter | 12 | 18.40 | 200 | 06.50 | 4 |
| Chipotle Ale | 12 | 17.10 | 173 | 05.40 | 3 |
| Chocolate Stout | 12 | 19.90 | 201 | 06.30 | 4 |
| Dead Guy | 12 | 22.10 | 216 | 06.60 | 4 |

| | Oz | Carbs | Cal | Abv | Weight Watcher's POINTS® |
|---|---|---|---|---|---|
| Double Dead Guy | 12 | 21.70 | 270 | 09.50 | 5 |
| Mocha Porter | 12 | 18.60 | 174 | 05.10 | 3 |
| Morimoto Imperial Pilsner | 12 | 17.30 | 240 | 08.80 | 5 |
| Morimoto Soba | 12 | 16.50 | 160 | 04.80 | 3 |
| Oregon Golden | 12 | 19.20 | 175 | 05.00 | 3 |
| Santa's Private Reserve | 12 | 13.70 | 171 | 06.00 | 3 |
| Shakespeare Stout | 12 | 21.50 | 202 | 06.00 | 4 |
| Smoke Ale | 12 | 20.00 | 195 | 05.90 | 4 |
| XS Imperial Stout | 12 | 40.60 | 366 | 10.50 | 7 |
| XS Old Crustacean | 12 | 31.60 | 346 | 11.30 | 7 |

**Rolling Rock**

| | Oz | Carbs | Cal | Abv | Weight Watcher's POINTS® |
|---|---|---|---|---|---|
| Extra Pale | 12 | 10.00 | 132 | 04.50 | 3 |
| Rock Light | 12 | 05.90 | 106 | 04.10 | 2 |

**SABMiller**

| | Oz | Carbs | Cal | Abv | Weight Watcher's POINTS® |
|---|---|---|---|---|---|
| 2M (Mozambique) | 12 | | 114 | 04.50 | 2 |
| Aguila (Columbia) | 12 | 12.78 | 135 | 03.80 | 3 |
| Arany Ászok (Hungary) | 12 | 09.94 | 131 | 04.50 | 3 |
| Arany Ászok Alkoholmentes (Hungary) | 12 | 10.65 | 053 | 00.50 | 1 |
| Atlas (Panama) | 12 | 08.88 | 110 | 03.70 | 2 |
| Balboa (Panama) | 12 | 11.00 | 135 | 04.50 | 3 |
| Birell (Czech Republic) | 12 | 14.20 | 067 | 00.50 | 1 |
| Carling Black Label (Botswana) | 12 | | 138 | 05.50 | 3 |
| Carling Black Label (Lesotho) | 12 | | 138 | 05.50 | 3 |

| | Oz | Carbs | Cal | Abv | Weight Watcher's POINTS® |
|---|---|---|---|---|---|
| Carling Black Label (Lesotho) | 12 | | 138 | 05.00 | 3 |
| Carling Black Label (South Africa) | 12 | | 138 | 05.50 | 3 |
| Carling Black Label (Swailand) | 12 | | 138 | 05.50 | 3 |
| Carling Black Label (Zimbabwe) | 12 | | 138 | 05.50 | 3 |
| Castle Lager (Botswana) | 12 | | 138 | 05.00 | 3 |
| Castle Lager (GB) | 12 | | 138 | 05.00 | 3 |
| Castle Lager (Lesotho) | 12 | | 138 | 05.00 | 3 |
| Castle Lager (South Africa) | 12 | | 138 | 05.00 | 3 |
| Castle Lager (Swaziland) | 12 | | 138 | 05.00 | 3 |
| Castle Lager (Tanzania) | 12 | | 138 | 05.00 | 3 |
| Castle Lager (Zambia) | 12 | | 138 | 05.00 | 3 |
| Castle Lager (Zimbabwe) | 12 | | 138 | 05.00 | 3 |
| Castle Milk Stout (Ghana) | 12 | | 178 | 06.00 | 3 |
| Ciucas (Romania) | 12 | | 135 | 04.50 | 3 |
| Club (Ecuador) | 12 | | 156 | 04.40 | 3 |
| Club Pilsner Lager (Uganda) | 12 | | 124 | 04.50 | 2 |
| Club Premium Lager (Ghana) | 12 | | 142 | 05.00 | 3 |
| Cristal (Peru) | 12 | 11.00 | 135 | 05.00 | 3 |

|  | Oz | Carbs | Cal | Abv | Weight Watcher's POINTS® |
|---|---|---|---|---|---|
| Cusqueña (Peru) | 12 | 11.00 | 142 | 05.00 | 3 |
| Dorada (Canary Islands) | 12 | 13.85 | 142 | 04.60 | 3 |
| Dorada (Ecuador) | 12 | 11.00 | 135 | 04.00 | 3 |
| Dorada Especial (Canary Islands) | 12 | 16.33 | 167 | 05.70 | 3 |
| Dorada Sin (Canary Islands) | 12 | 20.24 | 092 | 00.50 | 2 |
| Dreher Alkoholmentes (Hungary) | 12 | 10.65 | 053 | 00.50 | 1 |
| Dreher Classic (Hungary) | 12 | 11.00 | 149 | 05.20 | 3 |
| Eagle Lager Extra (Uganda) | 12 |  | 178 | 06.50 | 3 |
| Fosters (India) | 12 | 13.49 | 178 | 04.80 | 3 |
| Gambrinus 10 (Czech Republic) | 12 | 09.59 | 124 | 04.10 | 2 |
| Golden Light (El Salvador) | 12 | 07.46 | 114 | 04.00 | 2 |
| Hansa Pilsener (Botswana) | 12 |  | 114 | 04.50 | 2 |
| Hansa Pilsener (South Africa) | 12 |  | 114 | 04.50 | 2 |
| Hansa Pilsener (Swaziland) | 12 |  | 114 | 04.50 | 2 |
| Hansa Pilsner (Lesotho) | 12 |  | 114 | 04.50 | 2 |
| Imperial (Honduras) | 12 | 12.07 | 156 | 05.20 | 3 |
| Kilimanjaro Premium Lager (Tanzania) | 12 |  | 124 | 04.50 | 2 |
| Knock Out (India) | 12 | 13.85 | 192 | 07.20 | 4 |
| Kobanyai Sor (Hungary) | 12 | 09.59 | 128 | 04.50 | 2 |

| | Oz | Carbs | Cal | Abv | Weight Watcher's POINTS® |
|---|---|---|---|---|---|
| Kozel (Russia) | 12 | 12.07 | 128 | 03.70 | 2 |
| Kozel 10 (Czech Republic) | 12 | 06.75 | 117 | 04.00 | 2 |
| Lech (GB) | 12 | 09.59 | 146 | 05.20 | 3 |
| Lech Free (Poland) | 12 | 22.37 | 103 | 00.50 | 2 |
| Lech Premium (Poland) | 12 | 09.59 | 146 | 05.20 | 3 |
| Lion Lager (Zimbabwe) | 12 | | 181 | 04.90 | 4 |
| Malta (Tanzania) | 12 | | 209 | 00.00 | 4 |
| Manica (Mozambique) | 12 | | 131 | 05.00 | 3 |
| Miller Genuine Draft (GB) | 12 | 13.14 | 142 | 04.70 | 3 |
| Miller Genuine Draft (USA) | 12 | 13.10 | 143 | 04.70 | 3 |
| Miller High Life (USA) | 12 | 13.10 | 143 | 04.70 | 3 |
| Miller Lite (USA) | 12 | 03.20 | 096 | 04.20 | 2 |
| Mosi Lager (Zamia) | 12 | 08.88 | 131 | 04.00 | 3 |
| N'gola (Angola) | 12 | | 138 | 05.00 | 3 |
| Nile Special Lager (Uganda) | 12 | | 153 | 05.60 | 3 |
| Peroni (Italy) | 12 | 11.00 | 138 | 04.70 | 3 |
| Peroni Gran Riserva (GB) | 12 | 14.91 | 195 | 06.60 | 4 |
| Peroni Nastro Azzurro (GB) | 12 | 11.72 | 149 | 05.10 | 3 |
| Peroni Nastro Azzurro (Italy) | 12 | 11.72 | 149 | 05.10 | 3 |
| Peroni Red (GB) | 12 | 15.62 | 170 | 05.20 | 3 |

| | Oz | Carbs | Cal | Abv | Weight Watcher's POINTS® |
|---|---|---|---|---|---|
| Pilsen (Columbia) | 12 | 11.72 | 163 | 04.20 | 3 |
| Pilsen Callao (Peru) | 12 | 11.00 | 135 | 05.00 | 3 |
| Pilsener (Ecuador) | 12 | 11.72 | 138 | 04.20 | 3 |
| Pilsener (El Salvador) | 12 | 10.30 | 135 | 04.50 | 3 |
| Pilsner Urquell (GB) | 12 | 16.69 | 149 | 04.40 | 3 |
| Pilsner Urquell 12 (Czech Republic) | 12 | 16.69 | 149 | 04.40 | 3 |
| Poker (Columbia) | 12 | 12.78 | 135 | 03.90 | 3 |
| Pony Malta (Columbia) | 12 | | 160 | 00.00 | 3 |
| Pony Malta (Ecuador) | 12 | | 160 | 00.00 | 2 |
| Port Royal (Honduras) | 12 | 11.72 | 153 | 04.90 | 3 |
| Redd's (Vietnam) | 12 | | 138 | 04.20 | 3 |
| Regia Extra (El Salvador) | 12 | 12.07 | 156 | 05.30 | 3 |
| Royal Challenge (India) | 12 | 11.72 | 135 | 04.90 | 3 |
| Safari Lager (Tanzania) | 12 | | 146 | 05.50 | 3 |
| Salva Vida (Honduras) | 12 | 11.72 | 149 | 04.80 | 3 |
| Saris 10° (Slovakia) | 12 | 06.39 | 131 | 04.10 | 3 |
| Smadny Mnich 10° | 12 | 07.46 | 131 | 04.30 | 3 |
| Snow (11P) (China) | 12 | | 138 | 04.70 | 3 |
| Snow (8P) (China) | 12 | | 099 | 03.40 | 2 |
| Snow (9P) (China) | 12 | | 114 | 03.80 | 2 |
| Sterling Light Lager (South Africa) | 12 | | 110 | 02.50 | 2 |

|  | Oz | Carbs | Cal | Abv | Weight Watcher's POINTS® |
|---|---|---|---|---|---|
| Timisorena (Romania) | 12 | 11.36 | 149 | 05.00 | 3 |
| Topvar (Slovakia) | 12 | 10.65 | 124 | 04.10 | 2 |
| Tourtel (Italy) | 12 | 22.37 | 096 | 00.40 | 2 |
| Tropical (Canary Islands) | 12 | 13.85 | 142 | 04.60 | 3 |
| Tropical Sin (Canary Islands) | 12 | 20.24 | 092 | 00.50 | 2 |
| Tyskie (GB) | 12 | 10.65 | 153 | 05.60 | 3 |
| Tyskie (Poland) | 12 | 10.65 | 153 | 05.60 | 3 |
| Ursus (Romania) | 12 | 10.30 | 149 | 05.30 | 3 |
| Velkopopovicky Kozel 10° (Slovakia) | 12 | 06.75 | 117 | 04.00 | 2 |
| Vitamalt-Plus (Ghana) | 12 | 57.16 | 245 | 00.00 | 5 |
| Wuhrer/Raffo (Italy) | 12 | 11.00 | 138 | 04.70 | 3 |
| Zolotaya Bochka Classic (Russia) | 12 | 14.20 | 160 | 05.00 | 3 |
| Zolotaya Bochka Svetloe (Russia) | 12 | 16.33 | 149 | 04.00 | 3 |
| Zorok Lager Beer (Vietnam) | 12 |  | 142 | 05.00 | 3 |
| Zubur (Poland) | 12 | 11.36 | 174 | 06.00 | 3 |

### Sainsbury (UK)

|  | Oz | Carbs | Cal | Abv | Weight Watcher's POINTS® |
|---|---|---|---|---|---|
| Diät Pils | 500 ml | 02.85 | 190 | 06.20 | 4 |

### Saint Arnold

|  | Oz | Carbs | Cal | Abv | Weight Watcher's POINTS® |
|---|---|---|---|---|---|
| Amber Ale | 12 | 18.10 | 178 | 05.50 | 3 |
| Brown Ale | 12 | 17.00 | 171 | 05.30 | 3 |
| Christmas Ale | 12 | 21.20 | 220 | 07.00 | 4 |
| Divine Reserve | 12 | 20.50 | 245 | 08.40 | 5 |

| | Oz | Carbs | Cal | Abv | Weight Watcher's POINTS® |
|---|---|---|---|---|---|
| Elissa IPA | 12 | 18.00 | 200 | 06.60 | 4 |
| Fancy Lawnmower | 12 | 12.90 | 147 | 04.90 | 3 |
| Oktoberfest | 12 | 21.40 | 202 | 06.00 | 4 |
| Spring Bock | 12 | 21.90 | 212 | 06.40 | 4 |
| Summer Pils | 12 | 17.50 | 165 | 04.90 | 3 |
| Texas Treat | 12 | 16.60 | 162 | 04.90 | 3 |
| Winter Stout | 12 | 23.70 | 203 | 05.60 | 4 |

## Saku (Estonia)

| | Oz | Carbs | Cal | Abv | |
|---|---|---|---|---|---|
| Kuld | 12 | 11.00 | 142 | 04.50 | 3 |
| Originaal | 12 | 10.65 | 160 | 04.60 | 3 |

## Santa Fe

| | Oz | Carbs | Cal | Abv | |
|---|---|---|---|---|---|
| Barley Wine | 12 | 28.60 | 307 | 10.00 | 6 |
| Belgian | 12 | 19.20 | 221 | 07.50 | 4 |
| IPA | 12 | 25.50 | 225 | 06.30 | 4 |
| Nut Brown | 12 | 18.40 | 174 | 05.20 | 3 |
| Pale Ale | 12 | 20.60 | 189 | 05.50 | 4 |
| Pilsner | 12 | 20.60 | 189 | 05.50 | 4 |
| Porter | 12 | 27.40 | 206 | 05.00 | 4 |
| Stout | 12 | 17.30 | 167 | 05.00 | 3 |
| Wheat | 12 | 18.40 | 174 | 05.25 | 3 |

## Sapporo (Japan)

| | Oz | Carbs | Cal | Abv | |
|---|---|---|---|---|---|
| Premium | 12 | 10.30 | 140 | 04.90 | 3 |
| Premium Light | 12 | 08.50 | 119 | 03.99 | 2 |
| Reserve | 12 | 11.40 | 151 | 05.00 | 3 |

## Saxer

| | Oz | Carbs | Cal | Abv | |
|---|---|---|---|---|---|
| Bock | 12 | 23.80 | 217 | 06.30 | 4 |
| Dark Bock | 12 | 19.30 | 170 | 05.70 | 3 |
| Lemon Lager | 12 | 14.50 | 150 | 03.80 | 3 |

| | Oz | Carbs | Cal | Abv | Weight Watcher's POINTS® |
|---|---|---|---|---|---|
| Pilsner | 12 | 15.30 | 168 | 05.50 | 3 |
| Winter Doppelbock | 12 | 24.90 | 244 | 07.10 | 5 |

## Schlafly

| | Oz | Carbs | Cal | Abv | Weight Watcher's POINTS® |
|---|---|---|---|---|---|
| Coffee Stout | 12 | 19.00 | 195 | 05.70 | 4 |
| Pale Ale | 12 | 16.50 | 155 | 04.40 | 3 |
| Hefeweizen | 12 | 13.50 | 125 | 03.90 | 2 |
| Oatmeal Stout | 12 | 19.00 | 195 | 05.70 | 4 |
| Oktoberfest | 12 | 22.20 | 185 | 05.10 | 4 |
| Pilsner | 12 | 18.00 | 170 | 04.80 | 3 |
| Raspberry Hefe | 12 | 12.60 | 125 | 03.90 | 2 |
| Summer Kolsch | 12 | 15.50 | 160 | 04.80 | 3 |

## Scottish & Newcastle (Scotland)

| | Oz | Carbs | Cal | Abv | Weight Watcher's POINTS® |
|---|---|---|---|---|---|
| McEwans Scotch Ale | 12 | | 295 | 09.50 | 6 |

## Shipyard

| | Oz | Carbs | Cal | Abv | Weight Watcher's POINTS® |
|---|---|---|---|---|---|
| Export Ale | 12 | 12.00 | 141 | 05.10 | 3 |
| IPA | 12 | 13.33 | | | |
| Light | 12 | 07.40 | 097 | 03.20 | 2 |
| Old Thumper | 12 | 13.70 | 157 | 05.80 | 3 |
| Pumpkinhead Ale | 12 | 10.80 | | | |
| SeaDog Bluepaw | 12 | 10.80 | | | |
| Summer Ale | 12 | 12.20 | | | |

## Sierra Nevada

| | Oz | Carbs | Cal | Abv | Weight Watcher's POINTS® |
|---|---|---|---|---|---|
| Anniversary | 12 | 17.30 | 190 | 05.90 | 4 |
| Bigfoot | 12 | 32.10 | 330 | 09.60 | 7 |
| Celebration | 12 | 19.40 | 214 | 06.80 | 4 |
| Draft Ale | 12 | 13.40 | 157 | 05.00 | 3 |
| Early Spring | 12 | 16.70 | 190 | 05.90 | 4 |

| | Oz | Carbs | Cal | Abv | Weight Watcher's POINTS® |
|---|---|---|---|---|---|
| Harvest | 12 | 19.30 | 215 | 06.70 | 4 |
| IPA | 12 | 20.00 | 231 | 06.90 | 5 |
| Pale Ale | 12 | 14.10 | 175 | 05.60 | 3 |
| Pale Bock | 12 | 19.70 | 218 | 07.00 | 4 |
| Porter | 12 | 18.40 | 194 | 05.60 | 4 |
| Stout | 12 | 22.30 | 225 | 05.80 | 4 |
| Summerfest | 12 | 13.70 | 158 | 05.00 | 3 |
| Wheat | 12 | 13.10 | 153 | 04.40 | 3 |

## Silver City

| | Oz | Carbs | Cal | Abv | |
|---|---|---|---|---|---|
| Oktoberfest | 12 | 21.00 | 192 | 05.60 | 4 |
| Sasquatch Stout | 12 | 21.30 | 214 | 06.60 | 4 |
| Winter Bock | 12 | 22.50 | 224 | 06.90 | 4 |

## Silver Gulch

| | Oz | Carbs | Cal | Abv | |
|---|---|---|---|---|---|
| Amber Ale | 12 | 19.20 | 186 | 05.70 | 4 |
| Lager | 12 | 18.10 | 180 | 05.60 | 4 |
| Pilsner | 12 | 16.50 | 177 | 05.70 | 3 |
| Porter | 12 | 28.30 | 220 | 05.50 | 4 |

## Sinebrychoff (Russia)

| | Oz | Carbs | Cal | Abv | |
|---|---|---|---|---|---|
| 4.1 Täyteläinen Keyt Olut | 12 | 04.97 | 107 | 04.10 | 2 |
| Amiraali III | 12 | 08.52 | 124 | 04.30 | 2 |
| Carlsberg III | 12 | 08.17 | 142 | 04.50 | 3 |
| Carlsberg IVA | 12 | 09.23 | 142 | 05.00 | 3 |
| Carlsberg Lite | 12 | 01.42 | 089 | 04.10 | 2 |
| Jacobsen Extra | 12 | 16.33 | 192 | 05.50 | 4 |
| Jouluolut III | 12 | 15.98 | 160 | 04.60 | 3 |
| Jouluolut IV | 12 | 13.14 | 178 | 06.00 | 3 |
| Karhu III | 12 | 09.23 | 142 | 04.60 | 3 |

|  | Oz | Carbs | Cal | Abv | Weight Watcher's POINTS® |
|---|---|---|---|---|---|
| Karhu A | 12 | 11.36 | 160 | 05.30 | 3 |
| Koff I | 12 | 11.00 | 107 | 02.50 | 2 |
| Koff III | 12 | 07.81 | 142 | 04.50 | 2 |
| Koff IV A | 12 | 10.65 | 160 | 05.20 | 3 |
| Koff IV B | 12 | 12.43 | 213 | 07.50 | 4 |
| Koff Indian Beer | 12 | 07.81 | 124 | 04.40 | 3 |
| Koff Lite | 12 | 03.78 | 089 | 04.20 | 2 |
| Light | 12 | 05.33 | 107 | 04.10 | 2 |
| NA Nikolai | 12 | 10.30 | 053 | 00.00 | 1 |
| NA Nikolai Tumma | 12 | 13.14 | 064 | 00.00 | 1 |
| Nikolai Premium | 12 | 16.33 | 160 | 04.50 | 3 |
| Nikolai Tumma | 12 | 16.69 | 160 | 04.50 | 3 |
| Nikolai III | 12 | 16.69 | 160 | 04.50 | 3 |
| Nikolai IVA | 12 | 17.75 | 195 | 05.50 | 4 |
| Nikolai 0.0% | 12 | 10.30 | 053 | 00.00 | 1 |
| Perhekalja | 12 | 07.81 | 089 | 02.20 | 2 |
| Perrinnekalja | 12 | 08.17 | 089 | 02.20 | 2 |
| Saku Originaal | 12 | 10.65 | 160 | 04.60 | 3 |
| Sinebrychoff Porter | 12 | 17.04 | 231 | 07.20 | 5 |
| Special Strength | 12 | 11.36 | 213 | 08.00 | 4 |
| Tosi Vahva Karhu | 12 | 11.00 | 213 | 08.00 | 4 |
| Tuborg Classic | 12 | 09.23 | 142 | 04.50 | 3 |
| Velvet | 12 | 12.43 | 160 | 04.70 | 3 |

### Singha (Thailand)

| | Oz | Carbs | Cal | Abv | |
|---|---|---|---|---|---|
| Singha Light | 12 | 07.86 | 096 | 03.50 | 2 |

### Skagit River

| | Oz | Carbs | Cal | Abv | |
|---|---|---|---|---|---|
| Brown Ale | 12 | 16.60 | 193 | 06.50 | 4 |

| | Oz | Carbs | Cal | Abv | Weight Watcher's POINTS® |
|---|---|---|---|---|---|
| Delrio | | | | | |
| American Lager | 12 | 09.95 | 117 | 03.90 | 2 |
| Dutch Girl Lager | 12 | 13.40 | 157 | 05.30 | 3 |
| Highwater Porter | 12 | 21.25 | 230 | 07.50 | 5 |
| Scullers | 12 | 17.50 | 212 | 07.30 | 4 |
| Washington's Wheat Ale | 12 | 13.50 | 145 | 04.50 | 3 |
| Yellowjacket Pale Ale | 12 | 12.50 | 144 | 04.70 | 3 |

## Sleeman

| | Oz | Carbs | Cal | Abv | POINTS |
|---|---|---|---|---|---|
| Clear | 12 | 02.50 | 090 | 04.00 | 2 |
| Premium Light | 12 | | 095 | 04.00 | 2 |

## Smirnoff (Malt-Based)

| | Oz | Carbs | Cal | Abv | POINTS |
|---|---|---|---|---|---|
| Ice Arctic Berry | 12 | 38.30 | 248 | 05.00 | 5 |
| Ice Black Cherry | 12 | 38.00 | 238 | 05.00 | 5 |
| Ice Green Apple Bite | 12 | 40.50 | 252 | 05.00 | 5 |
| Ice Light | 12 | 08.50 | 099 | 03.20 | 2 |
| Ice Mandarin Orange | 12 | 35.90 | 231 | 05.00 | 5 |
| Ice Pomegranate Fusion | 12 | 35.90 | 241 | 05.00 | 5 |
| Ice Raspberry Burst | 12 | 38.30 | 245 | 05.00 | 5 |
| Ice FMB | 12 | 38.00 | 206 | 03.20 | 4 |
| Ice Watermelon | 12 | 35.50 | 238 | 05.00 | 5 |
| Ice Wild Grape | 12 | 36.90 | 241 | 05.00 | 5 |
| Raw Tea Green | 12 | 32.70 | 227 | 05.00 | 5 |
| Raw Tea Lemon | 12 | 37.60 | 234 | 05.00 | 5 |
| Raw Tea Raspberry | 12 | 32.00 | 227 | 05.00 | 5 |
| Source | 12 | 14.20 | 124 | 03.50 | 3 |
| Triple Black FMB | 12 | 36.60 | 241 | 05.00 | 5 |

|  | Oz | Carbs | Cal | Abv | Weight Watcher's POINTS® |
|---|---|---|---|---|---|
| Twisted V Black Cherry | 12 | 35.50 | 170 | 03.20 | 3 |
| Twisted V Black Cherry | 12 | 37.30 | 238 | 05.00 | 5 |
| Twisted V Green Apple | 12 | 39.80 | 213 | 03.20 | 4 |
| Twisted V Mandarin Orange | 12 | 40.10 | 252 | 03.20 | 5 |
| Twisted V Mandarin Orange | 12 | 35.90 | 231 | 05.00 | 4 |
| Twisted V Raspberry | 12 | 40.10 | 217 | 03.20 | 4 |
| Twisted V Raspberry | 12 | 40.10 | 245 | 05.00 | 5 |
| Twisted V Watermelon | 12 | 36.20 | 238 | 05.00 | 5 |
| Twisted V Wild Grape | 12 | 35.90 | 238 | 05.00 | 5 |

## Smithwick's (UK)

|  | Oz | Carbs | Cal | Abv | POINTS |
|---|---|---|---|---|---|
| Bottle | 12 | 07.10 | 128 | 04.50 | 2 |
| Draught | 12 | 07.10 | 128 | 04.50 | 2 |

## Snipes Mountain

|  | Oz | Carbs | Cal | Abv | POINTS |
|---|---|---|---|---|---|
| American Hefeweizen | 12 | 13.20 | 138 | 04.30 | 3 |
| Coyote Moon | 12 | 17.90 | 148 | 03.90 | 3 |
| Extra Blonde Ale | 12 | 15.70 | 146 | 04.30 | 3 |
| Harvest Ale | 12 | 18.60 | 174 | 05.10 | 3 |
| IPA | 12 | 21.70 | 196 | 05.60 | 4 |
| Porter | 12 | 22.70 | 170 | 04.15 | 3 |
| Roza Reserve | 12 | 33.30 | 312 | 09.20 | 6 |
| Sunnyside Pale Ale | 12 | 19.60 | 168 | 04.60 | 3 |

## Spaten-Brau (Germany)

|  | Oz | Carbs | Cal | Abv | POINTS |
|---|---|---|---|---|---|
| Lager | 12 |  | 150 | 05.20 | 3 |

| | Oz | Carbs | Cal | Abv | Weight Watcher's POINTS® |
|---|---|---|---|---|---|
| **Munich Special Dark Beer** | 12 | | 185 | 06.60 | 4 |
| **Spoetzl** | | | | | |
| Shiner Blond | 12 | 12.40 | 140 | 04.40 | 3 |
| Shiner Bock | 12 | 12.50 | 143 | 04.40 | 3 |
| Shiner Dunkelweizen | 12 | 19.60 | 193 | 05.40 | 4 |
| Shiner Leicht | 12 | 04.70 | 099 | 04.40 | 2 |
| Shiner Light | 12 | 09.10 | 120 | 04.00 | 2 |
| Shiner Summer Stock | 12 | 13.50 | 150 | 03.85 | 3 |
| **Sprecher** | | | | | |
| Abbey Triple | 12 | 23.80 | 258 | 08.41 | 5 |
| Barley Wine | 12 | 41.10 | 352 | 09.71 | 7 |
| Black Bavarian | 12 | 23.70 | 204 | 05.85 | 4 |
| Dopple Bock | 12 | 27.10 | 260 | 07.85 | 5 |
| Generation Porter | 12 | 19.10 | 188 | 05.75 | 4 |
| Hefe Weiss | 12 | 16.20 | 147 | 04.20 | 3 |
| IPA² | 12 | 22.70 | 257 | 07.50 | 5 |
| Irish Stout | 12 | 19.30 | 188 | 05.75 | 4 |
| Light | 12 | 14.70 | 135 | 04.16 | 3 |
| Maibock | 12 | 21.50 | 202 | 06.00 | 4 |
| Mbege (Gluten-Free) | 12 | 19.20 | 178 | 05.20 | 3 |
| Oktoberfest | 12 | 19.10 | 188 | 05.75 | 4 |
| Piper's Scotch Ale | 12 | 20.70 | 242 | 08.25 | 5 |
| Pub Ale | 12 | 18.40 | 161 | 04.50 | 3 |
| Russian Imperial Stout | 12 | 27.00 | 273 | 08.50 | 5 |
| Shakparo (Gluten -Free) | 12 | 19.30 | 188 | 05.70 | 4 |

|  | Oz | Carbs | Cal | Abv | Weight Watcher's POINTS® |
|---|---|---|---|---|---|
| Special Amber | 12 | 19.3 | 175 | 05.00 | 3 |
| Winter Brew | 12 | 21.10 | 195 | 05.75 | 4 |
| **St. Peter's (UK)** | | | | | |
| Summer Ale | 12 | 20.00 | 207 | 06.50 | 4 |
| **Stampede** | | | | | |
| Stampede Light | 12 | 08.80 | 115 | 03.80 | 2 |
| **Staropramen (Czech)** | | | | | |
| Dark | 12 | 12.78 | 142 | 04.40 | 3 |
| **Stoudt** | | | | | |
| Mai Bock | 12 | | 241 | 08.30 | 5 |
| **Straub** | | | | | |
| Straub | 12 | 10.10 | 128 | 04.33 | 2 |
| Straub Light | 12 | 07.16 | 096 | 03.16 | 2 |
| **Summit** | | | | | |
| Extra Pale Ale | 12 | 15.10 | 162 | 05.30 | 3 |
| Extra Special Bitter | 12 | 18.50 | 172 | 05.10 | 3 |
| Great Northern Porter | 12 | 18.30 | 182 | 05.60 | 4 |
| Hefe Weizen | 12 | 25.70 | 198 | 04.90 | 4 |
| IPA | 12 | 16.40 | 190 | 06.40 | 4 |
| Maibock | 12 | 22.20 | 218 | 06.70 | 4 |
| Oktoberfest | 12 | 18.90 | 219 | 07.40 | 4 |
| Pilsener | 12 | 13.40 | 151 | 05.10 | 3 |
| Scandia Ale | 12 | 17.40 | 163 | 04.80 | 3 |
| Winter Ale | 12 | 18.90 | 196 | 06.20 | 4 |
| **Suntory (Japan)** | | | | | |
| Draft Beer | 12 | | 138 | 04.60 | 3 |

| | Oz | Carbs | Cal | Abv | Weight Watcher's POINTS® |
|---|---|---|---|---|---|
| **Swashbuckler** | | | | | |
| Lady Amber Ale | 12 | 14.70 | 154 | 04.90 | 3 |
| Old Peg Leg Stout | 12 | 20.40 | 195 | 05.90 | 4 |
| Rajah's Sword Pale Ale | 12 | 21.30 | 183 | 05.10 | 4 |
| Scottland Strong Ale | 12 | 27.00 | 257 | 07.70 | 5 |
| Swashbuckler's Gold | 12 | 12.60 | 156 | 05.50 | 3 |
| **Terminal Gravity** | | | | | |
| Bar X Stout | 12 | 16.70 | 195 | 06.60 | 4 |
| Breakfast Porter | 12 | 22.00 | 197 | 05.70 | 4 |
| ESG | 12 | 11.60 | 150 | 05.40 | 3 |
| Festivale | 12 | 18.50 | 234 | 08.30 | 5 |
| IPA | 12 | 17.00 | 202 | 06.90 | 4 |
| **The Lion Brewery, Inc.** | | | | | |
| Lionshead | 12 | 13.20 | 138 | 04.40 | 3 |
| Lionshead Light | 12 | 10.00 | 117 | 04.00 | 2 |
| Little Kings | 12 | 14.50 | 170 | 05.40 | 3 |
| Pocono Amber Ale | 12 | 16.90 | 175 | 05.50 | 3 |
| Pocono Blonde Ale | 12 | 17.90 | 175 | 05.30 | 3 |
| Pocono Lager | 12 | 12.60 | 125 | 03.90 | 2 |
| Pocono Pale Ale | 12 | 17.50 | 185 | 06.00 | 4 |
| Stegmaier Amber Lager | 12 | 17.80 | 165 | 05.30 | 3 |
| Stegmaier Brewhouse Bock | 12 | 25.00 | 215 | 06.60 | 4 |
| Stegmaier Gold | 12 | 12.40 | 137 | 04.50 | 3 |
| Stegmaier Midsummer White | 12 | 17.50 | 170 | 04.90 | 3 |
| Stegmaier Oktoberfest | 12 | 18.50 | 188 | 05.90 | 4 |
| Stegmaier Porter | 12 | 22.40 | 175 | 04.40 | 3 |

|  | Oz | Carbs | Cal | Abv | Weight Watcher's POINTS® |
|---|---|---|---|---|---|
| Stegmaier Winter Warmer | 12 | 15.60 | 255 | 08.00 | 5 |
| **Three Floyds** | | | | | |
| Alpha King | 12 | 23.90 | 225 | 06.70 | 4 |
| Dreadnaught Imperial IPA | 12 | 32.10 | 316 | 09.70 | 6 |
| Gumballhead | 12 | 21.00 | 195 | 04.90 | 4 |
| Robert the Bruce | 12 | 24.30 | 231 | 06.90 | 5 |
| **Tinkoff (Russia)** | | | | | |
| Pilsner | 12 | 18.82 | 178 | 04.70 | 3 |
| Lager | 12 | 20.59 | 192 | 04.80 | 4 |
| Weissbier | 12 | 18.82 | 178 | 04.70 | 3 |
| Porter | 12 | 21.69 | 192 | 04.70 | 4 |
| Bock | 12 | 21.30 | 220 | 05.00 | 4 |
| **Tommyknocker Bewery & Pub** | | | | | |
| Butthead Bock | 12 | | 258 | 08.20 | 5 |
| **Trailhead** | | | | | |
| Missouri Brown Dark Ale | 12 | 19.75 | 182 | 05.30 | 4 |
| Old Courthouse Dry Stout | 12 | 16.40 | 159 | 04.80 | 3 |
| Riverboat Raspberry Fruit Ale | 12 | 14.40 | 148 | 04.70 | 3 |
| Trailblazer Blonde Ale | 12 | 11.35 | 131 | 04.40 | 3 |
| Trailhead Red Amber Ale | 12 | 18.90 | 166 | 04.70 | 3 |
| **Trumer (Austria)** | | | | | |
| Trumer Pils | 12 | 11.30 | 148 | 04.97 | 3 |

| | Oz | Carbs | Cal | Abv | Weight Watcher's POINTS® |
|---|---|---|---|---|---|
| **Tsingtao (China)** | | | | | |
| Tsingtao | 12 | 12.50 | 152 | 04.70 | 3 |
| Tsingtao Pure Draft | 12 | | 132 | 04.30 | 3 |
| **Tuborg (Denmark)** | | | | | |
| Tuborg Christmas | 12 | 16.80 | 166 | 05.10 | 3 |
| Tuborg Classic | 12 | 09.23 | 142 | 04.50 | 3 |
| Tuborg Gold | 12 | 16.33 | 163 | 05.00 | 3 |
| Tuborg Green | 12 | 16.33 | 149 | 04.60 | 3 |
| Tuborg Twist | 12 | 16.33 | 149 | 04.60 | 3 |
| **Two Brothers** | | | | | |
| Bitter End Pale Ale | 12 | 18.20 | 166 | 04.80 | 3 |
| Ebel's Weiss | 12 | 16.70 | 149 | 04.50 | 3 |
| Prairie Path Ale | 12 | 14.00 | 138 | 04.40 | 3 |
| Domaine Dupage | 12 | 23.10 | 206 | 05.90 | 4 |
| **Upland** | | | | | |
| Amber Ale | 12 | 19.70 | 189 | 05.70 | 4 |
| IPA | 12 | 18.70 | 207 | 06.80 | 4 |
| Pale Ale | 12 | 15.10 | 161 | 05.20 | 3 |
| Porter | 12 | 24.50 | 204 | 05.50 | 4 |
| Wheat | 12 | 22.10 | 176 | 04.50 | 3 |
| **Victory** | | | | | |
| Golden Monkey Tripel | 12 | 24.40 | 281 | 09.50 | 6 |
| HopDevil | 12 | 21.40 | 217 | 06.80 | 4 |
| Prima Pils | 12 | 16.30 | 171 | 05.50 | 3 |
| Storm King Stout | 12 | 27.60 | 286 | 09.10 | 6 |
| **Warsteiner (Germany)** | | | | | |
| Premium Fresh | 11.20 | 12.78 | 075 | <00.5 | 1 |

| | Oz | Carbs | Cal | Abv | Weight Watcher's POINTS® |
|---|---|---|---|---|---|
| Premium Verum | 12 | 10.60 | 150 | 04.80 | 3 |

## Weihenstephan (Germany)

| | Oz | Carbs | Cal | Abv | Weight Watcher's POINTS® |
|---|---|---|---|---|---|
| Fest | 12 | | 109 | 05.80 | 2 |
| Hefeweiss | 12 | 16.25 | 106 | 05.40 | 2 |
| Hefeweiss Dunkel | 12 | 17.00 | 104 | 05.30 | 2 |
| Korbinian | 12 | 25.25 | 161 | 07.40 | 3 |
| Kristall Weiss Bier | 12 | 16.25 | 109 | 05.40 | 2 |
| Original Lager | 12 | 13.75 | 102 | 05.10 | 2 |
| Vitus | 12 | | 123 | 07.70 | 2 |

## Wellhead

| | Oz | Carbs | Cal | Abv | Weight Watcher's POINTS® |
|---|---|---|---|---|---|
| Cisco Canyon Blonde | 12 | 13.40 | 157 | 05.30 | 3 |
| Crude Oil Stout | 12 | 20.00 | 173 | 04.80 | 3 |
| Indian Basin Wheat | 12 | 16.70 | 165 | 05.10 | 3 |
| Pale Ale | 12 | 13.40 | 157 | 05.30 | 3 |
| Roughneck Red | 12 | 17.20 | 171 | 05.30 | 3 |

## West Coast (New Zealand)

| | Oz | Carbs | Cal | Abv | Weight Watcher's POINTS® |
|---|---|---|---|---|---|
| Green Fern | 12 | 12.07 | 287 | 05.00 | 6 |

## Western Reserve

| | Oz | Carbs | Cal | Abv | Weight Watcher's POINTS® |
|---|---|---|---|---|---|
| Amber Ale | 12 | 19.20 | 185 | 05.60 | 4 |
| American Wheat | 12 | 14.90 | 173 | 05.90 | 3 |
| Bockzilla | 12 | 26.90 | 255 | 07.60 | 5 |
| Cloud Nine | 12 | 14.50 | 166 | 05.60 | 3 |
| McDamon's Irish | 12 | 17.90 | 206 | 06.90 | 4 |
| Nut Brown | 12 | 20.90 | 183 | 05.10 | 4 |
| Twist & Stout | 12 | 21.20 | 189 | 05.40 | 4 |
| Winter Ale | 12 | 26.20 | 248 | 07.40 | 5 |

## Widmer Brothers

| | Oz | Carbs | Cal | Abv | Weight Watcher's POINTS® |
|---|---|---|---|---|---|
| Alt | 12 | 13.60 | 160 | 04.90 | 3 |

| | Oz | Carbs | Cal | Abv | Weight Watcher's POINTS® |
|---|---|---|---|---|---|
| Blonde | 12 | 10.80 | 136 | 04.50 | 3 |
| Broken Halo IPA | 12 | 14.30 | 185 | 06.00 | 4 |
| Crimson Wheat | 12 | 16.50 | 184 | 04.90 | 4 |
| Dopplebock | 12 | 20.80 | 259 | 09.00 | 6 |
| Drop Top Amber Ale | 12 | 15.00 | 165 | 05.40 | 3 |
| Hefeweizen | 12 | 13.20 | 164 | 04.90 | 3 |
| HopJack | 12 | 14.80 | 184 | 05.00 | 4 |
| Northwest Red-Brrr | 12 | 18.00 | 230 | 07.15 | 5 |
| OKTŌ | 12 | 15.10 | 183 | 05.30 | 4 |
| Snow Plow Milk Stout | 12 | 31.00 | 237 | 05.50 | 5 |
| Sommerbraü | 12 | 10.20 | 154 | 04.80 | 3 |
| Summit Pale Ale | 12 | 18.40 | 187 | 05.73 | 4 |
| Widberry | 12 | 13.00 | 162 | 04.60 | 2 |
| Winternacht | 12 | 18.70 | 238 | 07.00 | 5 |

## Yellowstone Valley

| | Oz | Carbs | Cal | Abv | Weight Watcher's POINTS® |
|---|---|---|---|---|---|
| ESB | 12 | 19.50 | 191 | 05.90 | 4 |
| Huckle-Weizen | 12 | 15.20 | 164 | 05.30 | 3 |
| Oatmeal Stout | 12 | 19.50 | 191 | 05.90 | 4 |
| Wheat | 12 | 15.20 | 164 | 05.30 | 3 |
| Wild Fly Ale | 12 | 17.60 | 184 | 05.90 | 4 |

## Young's (UK)

| | Oz | Carbs | Cal | Abv | Weight Watcher's POINTS® |
|---|---|---|---|---|---|
| Chocolate Stout | 12 | 16.80 | | 05.20 | |
| Export Lager | 12 | 07.70 | | 05.00 | |
| Old Nick | 12 | 35.70 | | 07.20 | |
| Ram Rod | 12 | 12.25 | | 05.00 | |
| Special London Ale | 12 | 19.25 | | 06.40 | |

|  | Oz | Carbs | Cal | Abv | Weight Watcher's POINTS® |
|---|---|---|---|---|---|
| Waggledance Honey | 12 | 12.07 | 148 | 05.00 | 3 |
| Winter Warmer | 12 | 18.20 |  | 05.00 |  |

## Yazoo

|  | Oz | Carbs | Cal | Abv | Weight Watcher's POINTS® |
|---|---|---|---|---|---|
| Dos Perros | 12 | 18.10 | 140 | 03.50 | 3 |
| Hefeweizen | 12 | 15.30 | 159 | 05.00 | 3 |
| Pale Ale | 12 | 18.50 | 187 | 05.80 | 4 |
| Rye Porter | 12 | 20.70 | 194 | 05.70 | 4 |
| Stout | 12 | 19.70 | 153 | 03.80 | 3 |

## Yuengling

|  | Oz | Carbs | Cal | Abv | Weight Watcher's POINTS® |
|---|---|---|---|---|---|
| Premium | 12 | 12.00 | 150 | 04.40 | 3 |
| Light | 12 | 06.60 | 099 | 03.40 | 2 |
| Ale | 12 | 10.00 | 154 | 05.40 | 3 |
| Porter | 12 | 14.00 | 160 | 04.70 | 3 |
| Lager | 12 | 12.00 | 150 | 04.40 | 3 |
| Black & Tan | 12 | 14.00 | 155 | 04.70 | 3 |

Author Bob Skilnik is a certified brewer and 1991 alumnus of Chicago's Siebel Institute of Technology, the oldest brewing school in the United States, with a degree in Brewing Technology. He is also a former associate editor for the *American Breweriana Journal*; a contributor to various trade journals, magazines, and newspapers, including the *Chicago Tribune's* <u>Good Eating</u> section; and a frustrated former Chicago deli owner.

He has appeared on ABC's *The View*, the Fox News Channel's *Fox News Live*, ESPN2's *Cold Pizza* and WTTW's *Chicago Tonight* and scores of radio programs throughout the U.S., Canada and Europe as a beer authority.

Skilnik recently finished working with G. Bradley Publishing, Inc. in Saint Louis, Missouri and Chicago Public Television station WTTW as a contributor to a TV special and accompanying book, titled *Foods of Chicago: A Delicious History*. He is currently working on an illustrated book about the history of beer for Reaktion Book, Ltd. in London, England.

*Does My BUTT Look BIG In This BEER?* is his eighth book. The author has recently opened his own micro-publishing house, <u>Gambrinus Media</u>, which will specialize in working with authors with an interest in drink-related subjects. More information about manuscript submissions and publishing consulting can be found in the Spring of 2009 at http://www.BobSkilnik.com

LaVergne, TN USA
05 December 2010
207423LV00006B/90/P